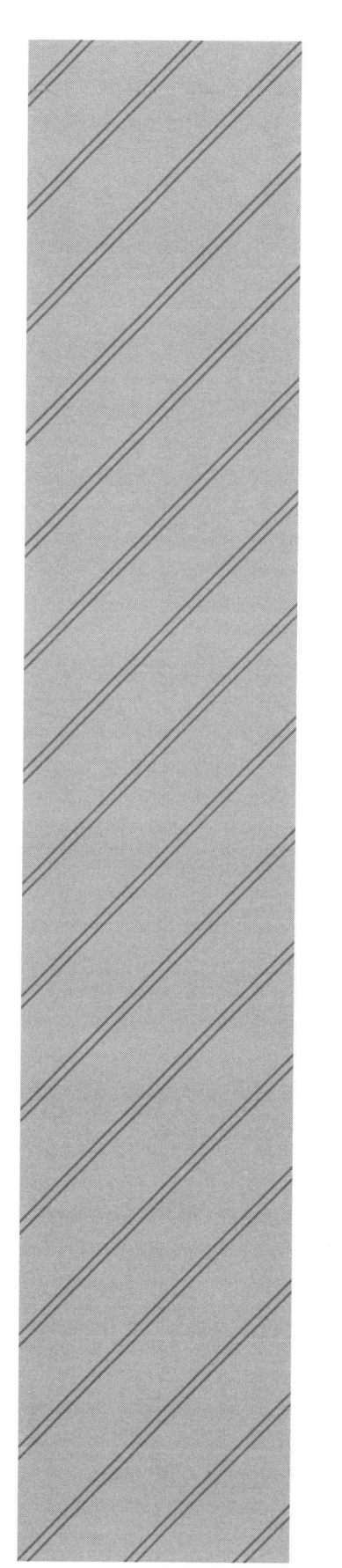

Teaching Kids About How AIDS Works

A Curriculum for Grades K–3

David J. Schonfeld, MD,
and Marcia Quackenbush, MS, MFCC

ETR ASSOCIATES
Santa Cruz, California
1996

ETR Associates (Education, Training and Research) is a nonprofit organization committed to fostering the health, well-being and cultural diversity of individuals, families, schools and communities. The publishing program of ETR Associates provides books and materials that empower young people and adults with the skills to make positive health choices. We invite health professionals to learn more about our high-quality publishing, training and research programs by contacting us at P.O. Box 1830, Santa Cruz, CA 95061-1830, (800) 321-4407.

About the Authors

David J. Schonfeld, MD, is a behavioral pediatrician and associate professor in the Department of Pediatrics and Child Study Center at Yale University School of Medicine, New Haven, Connecticut. He is the principal investigator of a 5-year study of young children's conceptual understanding of AIDS and the efficacy of school-based education at the elementary school level funded by the National Institute of Mental Health (MH47251). The results of the study have been published in *Pediatrics, AIDS Education and Prevention,* and the *Journal of Developmental and Behavioral Pediatrics* and have been reprinted in *Annual Progress in Child Psychiatry and Child Development 1994: A Selection of the Year's Outstanding Contributions to the Understanding and Treatment of the Normal and Disturbed Child.* He is known nationally and internationally for his work in pediatric bereavement, school-based crisis intervention and children's understanding of AIDS. He is an elected member of the Council of the International Society for HIV/AIDS Education and Prevention.

Marcia Quackenbush, MS, MFCC, is curriculum specialist and senior trainer at the AIDS Health Project, a program of the University of California, San Francisco. She has worked in the HIV field since 1984, and has provided direct services to a wide range of young people and adults facing HIV-related concerns. She has trained over 5,000 teachers, educators and health and mental health providers in HIV counseling and education. She is the coauthor of *Teaching AIDS* (ETR Associates, 1990), a resource guide for secondary school teachers; *Does AIDS Hurt? Educating Young Children About AIDS* (ETR Associates, 1992); *Risk and Recovery, AIDS, HIV and Alcohol* (AIDS Health Project, 1992), a handbook for providers; and *Handle with Care: Helping Children Prenatally Exposed to Drugs and Alcohol* (ETR Associates, 1992). She is a licensed marriage, family and child counselor in California and has a private practice in psychotherapy.

© 1996 by ETR Associates
All rights reserved. Published by ETR Associates,
P.O. Box 1830, Santa Cruz, CA 95061-1830

Permission to duplicate these materials is limited to the teacher for whom they are purchased. Reproduction for an entire school or school district is unlawful and strictly prohibited.

Printed in the United States of America

10 9 8 7 6 5 4 3 2

ISBN 1-56071-377-1

Text and cover design: Ann Smiley
Illustrations: Marcia Quackenbush

Title No. H421

Dedication

I would like to dedicate this book to my daughters, Sara and Kim, and the hundreds of children who participated in the research project that serves as the basis for this curriculum. They have shown me time and again that even young children are capable of understanding this illness and of demonstrating acceptance of and compassion for persons with AIDS.

—D.J.S.

Like David, I would like to dedicate this book to the children in my family and those who helped in the development of this curriculum. I want them to understand AIDS and to have confidence in their knowledge. I hope this book will play a role in helping younger children—my relatives and others—act with assurance as they mature, and protect themselves from HIV.

—M.Q.

This book is also dedicated to those who are infected by HIV and their families, friends and members of their community who are in turn affected. We join with them in the hope that one day we will no longer need to teach our children about AIDS.

Contents

Acknowledgments vii
Preface.. ix

Introduction 1
Why AIDS Education? 1
A Conceptually Based Approach 2
Differentiation: An Important Skill 2
Sequential Learning... 3
Involving Parents 3
Teacher Preparation... 4
A Special Note to Kindergarten Teachers 5
A Note About Language 5

What's in This Curriculum 7
The Units 7
Teacher Resource Section 9

The Curriculum: Activities for Students

Unit 1: **Different Illnesses** 13
    Activity 1—What Is Health? What Is Sickness? 16
    Activity 2—Different Illnesses 18
    Activity 3—If You're Sick, Can I Get It? 21
    Activity 4—Getting Help When I Am Sick 24
    Evaluation—How Illnesses Are Different....................26
    Family Activity 28

Unit 2: **Different Ways to Be Sick** 37
    Activity 1—What Is a Germ 40
    Activity 2—Seeing Is Believing: Watching "Germs" Pass 43
    Activity 3—Serious and Not-So-Serious Illnesses 46
    Evaluation—Elizabeth and Mrs. Shaw: A Story...........49
    Family Activity 51

Unit 3: **How the Body Stays Well** 59
    Activity 1—How Can Germs Get Inside the Body?....62
    Activity 2—The Body Protects Itself............................64
    Activity 3—Inside the Body: Defending the Castle ...66
    Activity 4—How Helper Cells Fight Germs................70
    Evaluation—The Immune System at Work 73
    Family Activity 73

Unit 4: What About AIDS? 79
    Activity 1—About AIDS 82
    Activity 2—Keeping "Inside" Germs Outside..................85
    Activity 3—How Is AIDS Passed?...................................88
    Activity 4—What Does the AIDS Germ Do to the Body? 93
    Evaluation—AIDS Is Hard to Get....................................96
    Family Activity 96

Unit 5: Preventing AIDS 101
    Activity 1—How Does AIDS Make People Sick 104
    Activity 2—Preventing AIDS 108
    Evaluation—What Kids Need to Know About AIDS.................110
    Family Activity 111

Unit 6: Helping Out 117
    Activity 1—Curriculum Review 120
    Activity 2—Guest Speaker, Film or Story 121
    Activity 3—Caring About People with AIDS
                and Their Families 122
    Activity 4—Making Cards 125
    Family Activity 126

For the Teacher: A Resource Section

Teacher Content Summaries..131

Review Guide..157

Information for Parents 160

Background Information About HIV 167

What Can Children Understand, When? 180

Guidelines for Discussing Sensitive Topics 186

Talking with Children About Death....................................193

Addressing Drug Use and AIDS 198

Selected Resources 200

Acknowledgments

We are appreciative of the outstanding efforts of Linda O'Hare as the research associate for the project and would like to gratefully acknowledge the assistance of the administration, staff and students of New Haven Public Schools who provided many of the ideas for the development of this curriculum, the opportunity to evaluate critically its effectiveness, and invaluable feedback during the evaluation process.

We would also like to thank our editor, Kay Clark. Her support and suggestions throughout the writing of this curriculum have helped us produce clearer language, better organization and a document we think teachers will be able to use easily. We have truly benefited from her dedication to the issue of AIDS education.

The following teachers and health educators provided valuable input in the early stages of the book's development:

Norma Dahnkin
McKinley Elementary School
San Francisco, California

Constanza Pedraza
Sunnyside Elementary School
San Francisco, California

Mickey Kavanagh
Hillhouse High School
New Haven, Connecticut

Nancy Charest
Hillhouse High School
New Haven, Connecticut

Patrice Flynn
Beecher Elementary School
New Haven, Connecticut

Karen Carazo
Beecher Elementary School
New Haven, Connecticut

Carol Westbrook
Marguerite Vann Elementary School
Conway, Arkansas

Lisa Unti
ETR Associates
Santa Cruz, California

Preface

THIS CURRICULUM WAS DEVELOPED out of a 5-year research project, funded by the National Institute of Mental Health, that sought to answer some essential questions about AIDS education and young children. First, what do elementary school children already know about AIDS and can we describe the processes by which they come to understand this illness? (This was the first phase of the project.)

Second, could children's conceptual knowledge about AIDS be advanced through classroom instruction? Or was their confusion and limited understanding the result of an age-appropriate developmental limitation. Certainly, teachers as well as parents know that as children grow and mature, they become able to understand and explore increasingly complex information. But is a young child's level of conceptual understanding fixed and unable to be changed by direct educational interventions?

Third, could factual knowledge about AIDS be taught and, if so, could children retain that knowledge over a period of time?

Fourth, could children be taught, and understand in a meaningful way, why they need not worry about getting HIV through casual contact?

And, finally, would this type of curriculum in any way increase children's anxiety about AIDS?

The answer to the first 4 questions was "yes." Students who participated in the project demonstrated successful learning of several important concepts about communicable diseases generally and about AIDS specifically. They retained their understanding over a period of time. The level of conceptual understanding they achieved was actually more sophisticated than some might have expected.

This leaves the question of anxiety. Were the lessons about AIDS disturbing to the children? The reassuring answer to this question was "no." Students who participated in the study did not show any increase in anxiety after receiving AIDS education.

What the Research Found

As part of the study, approximately 1,500 interviews were conducted with an ethnically diverse group of students (approximately 40% Black, 40% White and 20% Hispanic) attending kindergarten through sixth grade in New Haven [Connecticut] Public Schools. In the second phase of the study, this curriculum was presented to half the classes over a 3-week period.

Students in the other classes served as a comparison group.

A standardized, semi-structured interview was given to all students (including the comparison group) both before and after the intervention. The interview measured conceptual understanding, factual information and fears about AIDS.

Children who received the classroom intervention showed significant gains in their understanding of the causes of AIDS and ways AIDS is prevented. In fact, after the classroom intervention, students on average were able to demonstrate a level of understanding about the causes of AIDS that matched the sophistication of students 2 or more grades higher who had not received the curriculum. Student responses to open-ended questions in the interviews showed more accurate understanding and fewer misconceptions about the cause and prevention of AIDS than those students in the control group.

Most of these gains were still evident when the interview was repeated a third time, over 2 months later. Despite the considerable attention given to the subject over the course of the classroom lessons, children in the intervention group were no more likely to be afraid that they currently had AIDS, or would develop it in the future, than those in the control group.

A Theory-Based Curriculum

In the second phase of the study, all of the classroom teaching was provided by the principal investigator (David J. Schonfeld), a behavioral pediatrician with considerable knowledge of both children's cognitive development and AIDS. Understandably, there was some question about how students would do if taught by teachers with less expertise in these areas.

Therefore, in the third phase of the study, the teaching was provided by classroom teachers, who had received an inservice on AIDS and an orientation to the curriculum. The material in their training was no more indepth than what is made available here for users of this curriculum. The gains made by students in these classes were equivalent to those made by students in the second phase of the study.

The conclusion drawn from this encouraging finding is that the curriculum itself is the basis for success in this study. The curriculum's strengths include an emphasis on the learning and application of concepts rather than rote memorization of facts, repetition of concepts over time, and activities that actively engage children in new learning and the application of the concepts. The learning strategies do not rely on extraordinary expertise or other special capabilities on the part of the instructor, beyond what elementary classroom teachers already know about educating children.

This is the great benefit of a theory-based and empirically tested curriculum: It has a proven record of success with a number of students over a period of time, delivered by a range of instructors of varying levels of expertise and skill.

An AIDS-Specific Curriculum

Most educators recommend that AIDS education be integrated into a comprehensive health education program. Effective programs of this nature seek to promote health education that addresses the whole child—mentally, physically and socially. While it is appropriate and preferred to plan and sequence AIDS education into a larger program of this nature, we caution against curricula that attempt to be too global and that do not address the specific questions and concerns AIDS can raise among children.

Educational approaches that are very broad and general may suffer by being vague. School administrations that are apprehensive about the controversy raised by AIDS education may fall back on such approaches to avoid potential trouble. Teachers who are uncertain of their ability to teach about AIDS may find some solace in a more general and less specific treatment of the subject. Educators who question the need for AIDS education with children may even feel the broader, less candid type of lesson is a more appropriate route.

Children faced with such approaches are likely to find their misconceptions reinforced and their tendency to overgeneralize intensified. In this environment, they are unlikely to either advance their conceptual knowledge in any meaningful way, or to develop the cognitive skills necessary to evaluate past, current and future information about AIDS in a productive and effective manner. This is why a specific, sequenced AIDS curriculum, such as the one offered here, can be of such benefit to elementary-age students.

Introduction

Why AIDS Education?

AIDS is a serious illness, raises complex issues, and touches on controversial topics such as sexuality, drug use and death. Is it really necessary for children in early elementary grades to take on this subject?

The answer is straightforward and simple: Children have *already* received education about AIDS and HIV. They have heard about it on television and radio, among peers and older students, and in their families and communities. Unfortunately, because of the way much of this information makes its way to children, they have also acquired misunderstandings. The media in particular often aim to sensationalize or frighten, without truly educating. Children who receive incomplete and confusing messages may believe that AIDS is easily transmitted between people, as colds and flus are. In some research studies, many children expressed fears that they themselves had AIDS or would one day develop it.

Future projections in no way suggest that the AIDS epidemic is coming to a close. Rather, trends suggest that AIDS will become increasingly common in smaller cities and rural areas, and that the number of new cases of HIV will grow. Over time, more and more children will know someone who has HIV, or someone who has a family member, colleague or close friend affected by the virus. As it becomes increasingly common for children to know people affected by HIV, it will become increasingly important for children's misconceptions about AIDS to be addressed.

Today's early elementary students will grow to adulthood in a world where HIV is widespread. Thus, the behaviors they may engage in will present more significant dangers of HIV transmission. As early as fifth and sixth grade, some children will make decisions about drug experimentation, including injection drugs. Well before middle school, students in some areas report sexual activities among peers. As the prevalence of HIV increases in these communities, the risks of sexual or drug experimentation become considerable.

The issue facing teachers, schools and communities today is not whether to tell children about AIDS. Rather, it is whether steps will be taken to correct misconceptions, offer accurate information, and provide children with the concepts and skills they need to make sense of AIDS information now and in the future.

Children who receive accurate, clear, age-appropriate information are capable of learning important concepts about what AIDS is, how it is transmitted, how it can be prevented, and why it is not a common disease among children. This curriculum uses a number of effective strategies to help students achieve this learning.

A Conceptually Based Approach

Many AIDS curricula for young children, as well as those for middle and high school students, attempt simply to teach children facts about AIDS. Facts are often presented as isolated statements, without relation to underlying comprehension; for example, "AIDS is a serious disease, and many people have died of it." Children could memorize this or other facts easily, but unless facts can be applied in some practical way, they have little meaning.

Further, simply memorizing facts does not represent true learning. While the information can be parroted back, it cannot be applied to new situations, is not likely to change existing understanding, and, in many cases, is not remembered over time. Memorization in the absence of understanding is likely to be inaccurate and highly vulnerable to conflicting arguments, such as those offered by ill-informed peers, older students or sensationalistic media.

This curriculum uses a *conceptual basis* for delivery of information about AIDS, rather than a strictly factual approach. *Concepts* are broad statements that apply to a range of circumstances. Once children understand these concepts, they have a framework to help them evaluate and differentiate further information. For example, "There are different kinds of illnesses, and each illness makes people sick in different ways," is a concept that can help children *understand* that colds and AIDS are different kinds of illnesses. "Some diseases are serious, and others are not-so-serious," is a concept that can help children *understand* some of the specific ways AIDS is different from common colds and flus.

A conceptual approach to AIDS education helps students make sense of the facts they are taught, evaluate and correct past misunderstandings, and develop skills they can use to evaluate new information in the future.

Differentiation: An Important Skill

The single most important skill woven into the concepts in this curriculum is that of *differentiation*. Young children tend to overgeneralize new information. (See What Can Children Understand, When? p. 180.) This is normal, and very much in keeping with their developmental level. In AIDS education, this tendency can be seen in children's common concerns about a number of topics.

For example, children worry about casual transmission of AIDS because other diseases they know about, such as colds and flus, are easy to transmit. Therefore, they reason, AIDS must also be easy to transmit. Many children express concerns about their own susceptibility to AIDS. After all, they have heard on television that this dangerous and frightening disease is a risk for everyone. Understandably, some children assume they, their families and their schoolmates are likely to develop AIDS, probably sometime soon.

When children are taught the skills necessary to modify their tendency to overgeneralize, true comprehension of AIDS information can be achieved. For example, this curriculum begins with the concepts that different illnesses have different causes ("different ways someone gets them"), different symptoms ("each illness makes people sick in different ways") and different treatments ("there are different things people can do to get better from different illnesses"). As this foundation becomes established, children are better able to keep distinct their personal experiences about illnesses in general (usually common, easy-to-transmit and not serious in nature) and the new information they are learning about AIDS (uncommon among children, hard-to-transmit and very serious).

Sequential Learning

Units are presented in a specific and carefully designed sequence. Earlier units provide the foundation for later material. Students who do not gain a good grasp of the concepts in the first units may have difficulty in later units.

The first 3 units focus on communicable and non-communicable disease and offer students opportunities to build skills in differentiation (understanding that different illnesses have different causes, symptoms and treatments). Units 4 and 5 provide more specific information about AIDS. The final unit allows teachers to do a special project with the class as a way of marking the end of the series.

Involving Parents

Parents play a crucial role in AIDS education, from the elementary grades onward. An effective AIDS curriculum for children takes firm steps to welcome parent input and involve parents directly in their children's classroom experiences. For this reason, we encourage schools and teachers to place significant emphasis on the role parents can play in this educational process.

We suggest that parents receive a general notification letter describing the purpose and content of the curriculum before it is taught. This letter might include the rationale for providing the lessons, an outline of the material to be covered, and samples of actual teaching strategies. A sample letter is included in the Information for Parents section (p. 160). It is helpful to offer parents an opportunity to visit the school to preview the curriculum and discuss in person the material that will be taught and how certain topics will be handled.

Even if a school does not require parental consent or notification for AIDS education, a letter to parents is more than a simple courtesy. Children participating in an AIDS curriculum will have questions, and parents will want to be prepared for the kinds of questions their children may have. The Information for Parents section also includes a handout with basic information about HIV and AIDS to help parents feel more informed on the topic.

Additionally, in many circumstances, the preferred response to some of the children's questions will be to refer them back to their parents for further discussion. In some schools, this may be required when questions of an explicitly sexual nature are raised. But even in the most permissive teaching atmosphere, some questions will be most appropriately referred to parents. This is especially true of questions about values, morals and religious beliefs. If teachers know parents are prepared for these kinds of questions, they will feel much more comfortable making such referrals.

Many parents are very interested in an AIDS curriculum. Sometimes they will want to get their own questions about AIDS answered. Many will be grateful for the effort they see being put into this important element of their children's education. Teachers are sometimes quite pleasantly surprised at the positive feedback they receive from parents about the AIDS education process. When they understand exactly what is going on in the classroom, parents are less likely to become concerned, defensive or upset about the subject of AIDS being addressed in the school.

In this curriculum, parent letters are built into the family activity sheets that appear at the end of each unit. Family activity sheets include lesson objectives and concepts, as well as questions for parents to ask their children about what they have been studying. These family activities enable parents to participate in the lessons and confirm and reinforce what their children are learning in class.

Teacher Preparation

While no extraordinary expertise in the area of AIDS is required to implement the lessons in this curriculum, a basic understanding of the material will help teachers feel more confident about teaching the topic. The teacher resource section provides background information to supplement teacher knowledge and skills in areas unique to AIDS prevention education. It is suggested that teachers familiarize themselves with this material before beginning to implement the units.

Because every class will be different in terms of how much baseline knowledge students have about communicable disease, differences between illnesses, or the topic of AIDS itself, teachers can evaluate that material in a given unit for its usefulness for their students. They may elect to adjust the unit, presenting fewer activities overall, if students are already familiar with the concepts. However, since the concepts in this curriculum are both important and rich, it will not in any way hurt students to repeat and review earlier learning.

Because this is a curriculum designed for children spanning several years of development (kindergarten through third grade), teachers also will probably find it necessary to adjust the material to keep it at an appropriate level for their students. In general, the curriculum is written for an "average" second grade class. While the material is appropriate for children throughout the early elementary grades, certain predictable differences may emerge.

Third graders may be able to take discussions to more sophisticated levels; first graders may need help with prompts in discussions. Second graders might draw a picture showing what they have learned in the lesson, while third graders would draw a picture and write a short essay. Throughout the curriculum, suggestions for tailoring the material to more, or less, sophisticated students are offered.

It is important to evaluate students' understanding on an ongoing basis. With certain subjects, such as sexual transmission of HIV, special attention may be necessary to avoid aiming the level of the class to a few precocious students. Guidelines for Discussing Sensitive Topics (p. 186) offers suggestions for discussing sensitive issues in the classroom.

A Special Note to Kindergarten Teachers

While a range of maturity is evident in any elementary level class, this is often most striking with kindergarten students. Students who have been involved in preschool, daycare or Head Start programs may be well socialized, verbal, interactive and responsive to group activities. Children who have had little opportunity for socialization may not have experience discussing *any* topic in a group setting, much less something as complex as AIDS.

Additionally, kindergarten teachers will probably need to make the most adaptations in this curriculum, because the gap between their students' abilities and the content of the curriculum is probably greater than for other grades.

In the authors' experience teaching this curriculum, however, these youngest students did enjoy the lessons. Some of the content was more detailed than necessary, and some of the discussion questions were adapted and simplified. The demonstrations were effective and held the students' interest.

The authors' personal impression from working with kindergarten classes was that the lessons proved valuable and interesting to students. When students' responses were evaluated in the research portion of this project, the curriculum's ability to advance knowledge and comprehension about AIDS for kindergartners was comparable to students at other grade levels.

A Note About Language

There are some terms you will want to be familiar with as you use this curriculum.

AIDS: A disease that damages the immune system, making the person susceptible to a number of serious diseases that do not affect people with healthy immune systems.

HIV: *Human immunodeficiency virus*, the virus that causes AIDS. A person carrying the virus has HIV infection, sometimes called HIV disease, or simply HIV. A person may be infected with HIV for many years without signs or symptoms of illness.

People with HIV infection fall anywhere along a spectrum of illness:

- Some have no symptoms.
- Some have physical symptoms, but do not meet the criteria for an AIDS diagnosis.
- Some have physical symptoms and meet the criteria for an AIDS diagnosis.
- Some have no physical symptoms, but meet the criteria for an AIDS diagnosis.

Young children, especially those under age 7, generally will not make these distinctions between HIV and AIDS. They may ask questions about "AIDS," when the term "HIV infection" would be more accurate. This is also true of older children who have not had much exposure to information about HIV.

To keep explanations as simple as possible, we feel it is acceptable to sacrifice some points of scientific accuracy and keep the focus on more general concepts. This curriculum uses the terms "AIDS" and "the AIDS germ," or describes "people with the AIDS germ in their bodies" when providing information to children. In most cases, it has not been necessary to make the distinction between symptom-free HIV infection (at an early stage of illness) and someone with an AIDS diagnosis (at a later stage of illness).

You can assess the sophistication of your students and adapt the curriculum, using more accurate and specific terms if appropriate. Elementary-age children have certainly shown they are capable of understanding these differences. If your class enjoys learning new words or being precise in their language, you could spend some time clarifying terms like "HIV," "HIV infection," and "AIDS." Many children in AIDS-endemic areas, such as San Francisco, New Jersey, New York and Los Angeles, are likely to be familiar with this language already. However, the emphasis of the lessons should continue to be on understanding the general concepts (the AIDS germ is an "inside" germ, it is not easy to pass between people, it damages the body's ability to fight off other diseases), not on absolute accuracy of terminology.

What's in This Curriculum?

The Units

The 6 curriculum units are designed to be easy and practical to use. Student and family activity sheets are included behind each unit. Each unit contains the following features.

Objective Unit activities are designed to help students realize one overall unit objective. The last activity in each unit is an evaluation activity, intended to help teachers determine whether students satisfactorily achieved the unit objective.

In addition, a single specific learning objective is included for each activity within the unit. These activity objectives help lead students step-by-step to achievement of the overall unit objective.

Concepts The concepts listed at the beginning of each unit are the cornerstone of the curriculum—the conceptual basis for the lessons. Teachers are encouraged to read the concepts carefully, and think about the ways these concepts are taught in the activities of the unit. The goal is not for students to be able to parrot back the wording of the concepts, but to demonstrate skills in applying the concepts.

For example, a student who understands the concept, "There are some illnesses one person can catch from another, and some illnesses that one person cannot catch from another" (from Unit 1) will understand why he or she must avoid close contact with a best friend who has the flu, but can be close and affectionate with his or her grandmother who has had a stroke.

Time The overall time for the unit is given. In addition, time required for each activity is noted to help teachers plan.

How AIDS Works: Grades K–3

Overview   The overview provides a general rationale for the unit.

Unit Summary   The unit summary lists and briefly describes the activities for the unit, including evaluation and family activities.

Developmental Framework   This section offers suggestions for adapting the material for classes that may be a little less, or a little more, sophisticated than the level of the curriculum.

Terms to Use   Terms that are likely to be new for many students are listed in this section.

Review   Teacher Content Summaries are included for the units. These provide additional background information or suggestions for effective teaching. This section lists any content summaries that will be helpful preparation for the teacher.

Get Ready   Preparation steps for the unit are listed. This includes a list of any materials needed, student and family activity sheets that will need to be copied, and any special items that must be made by the teacher prior to presenting the unit.

Activities   The activities include detailed instructions that walk the teacher through the presentation. The activity objective is listed, as are the time needed, materials needed and any relevant Teacher Content Summaries.

At certain points in the activity steps, alternate approaches are suggested for younger students (working with less sophisticated information) and older students. Each class will be a little different in its interests, comprehension and pre-existing knowledge. Teachers are encouraged to select the approach that will be most useful for their individual class, whatever the grade level.

Ongoing assessment steps allow the teacher to assess student progress toward the objective.

Evaluation   The last activity in each unit is an evaluation activity designed to measure children's understanding of the unit concepts and achievement of the overall unit objective.

Family Activity   Each evaluation activity includes a special assignment to be sent home to families. Family activities enable parents to participate in the lessons and confirm and reinforce what children are learning in class.

Student Activity Sheets   The activity sheets used for classroom instruction or as homework exercises follow the activities. Sometimes, different materials are available for younger and older students. The materials for older students are more sophisticated; those for younger students are simpler.

Family Activity Sheets   Family activity sheets follow the student activity sheets. These sheets describe the content of the lessons and invite parents or guardians to discuss the classroom learning with their children.

Teacher Resource Section

The latter part of the book contains information for teachers. This resource section offers information to increase teachers' expertise and comfort level with special issues in HIV education.

Teacher Content Summaries   Teacher Content Summaries are included for each unit. These pages contain relevant background information and teaching suggestions to help teachers present the material in the various activities.

Review Guide   Reviewing concepts from previous units is an important component of this curriculum. This section provides questions and sample answers that can be used to review the main points presented in each unit.

Information for Parents

Parental support is critical to the success of any AIDS curriculum. This section offers guidelines for notifying parents and family members about the curriculum. It includes a sample parent notification letter to be sent home before the AIDS curriculum is implemented, as well as a handout with basic information about HIV and AIDS for parents.

Background Information About HIV

This section provides answers to many common questions about HIV and AIDS. It is intended to give teachers a foundation of general knowledge about the disease and the epidemic.

What Can Children Understand, When?

Information is provided to help teachers recognize the typical developmental stages children move through in their understanding of illnesses, death and sexuality.

Guidelines for Discussing Sensitive Topics

Teachers often have concerns about how to handle controversial subjects in the classroom. In addition, many schools and districts have policies governing which topics can be discussed in the school setting. This section offers suggestions for answering student questions around sensitive topics, to help teachers provide students with the information they need and deserve, yet adhere to school or district policies regarding controversial subject matter.

Talking with Children About Death

In discussions of AIDS, often the subject of death will arise. This article offers guidelines on addressing this sensitive topic with young children.

Addressing Drug Use and AIDS

Ideally, students will have already received instruction around drugs and drug use. This section offers a brief outline of what students should know about drugs and drug use before the lessons on AIDS are presented. The information is mainly a review of critical points and is not intended to be the only teaching students receive on drugs and drug use. (It is strongly recommended that a separate curriculum address the important subject of substance use in more depth.)

Selected Resources

An annotated resource list includes books and videos for children as well as general and specific resources for adults. Many of these can be used to supplement student understanding or help teachers prepare.

The Curriculum

Activities for Students

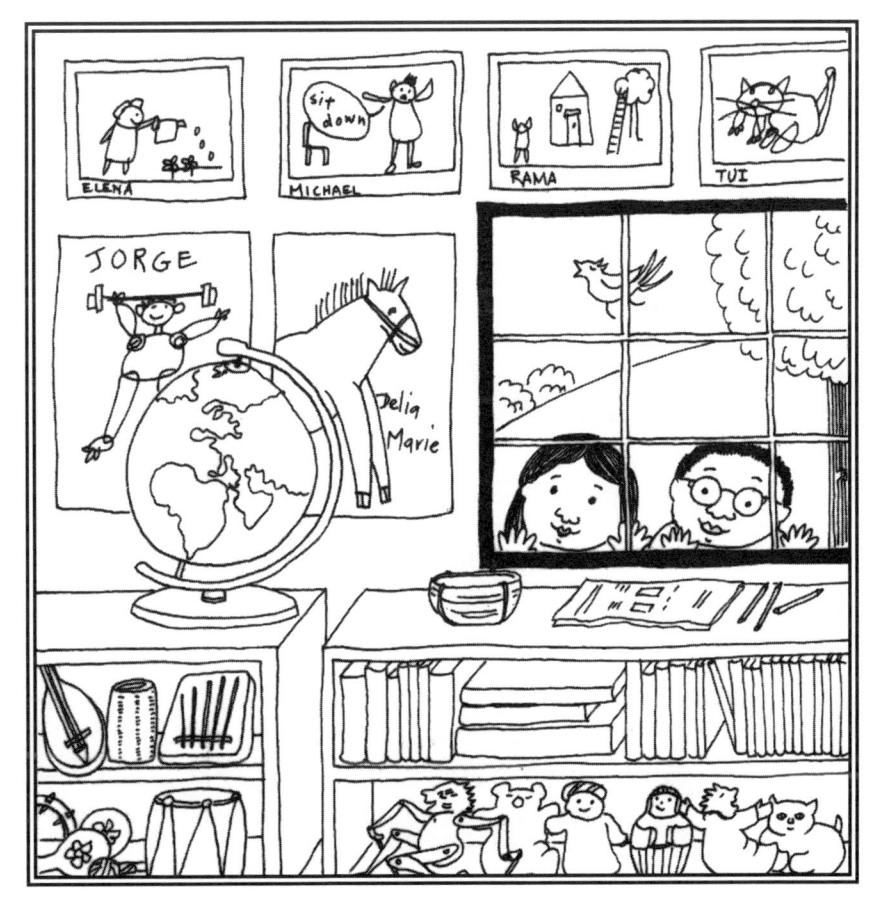

Unit 1

Different Illnesses

Time 75 minutes

Unit Objective Students will be able to describe 3 general ways illnesses differ from one another:

- There are different ways people get them.
- They have different symptoms.
- There are different ways to treat different illnesses.

Concepts
1. Everyone gets sick sometimes.
2. Different illnesses have different causes, different symptoms and different treatments.
3. There are some illnesses one person can catch from another (communicable), and some illnesses that one person cannot catch from another (non-communicable).

Overview Students probably already understand that illness is a normal part of life and that everyone gets sick sometimes. But young children tend to overgeneralize what they already know, which can lead to confusion and misunderstanding.

Any curriculum that addresses the serious illness of AIDS will be most successful when students have a foundation of knowledge in place that allows them to understand not only that AIDS is a "different kind of illness," but the reasons *why* it is different.

(continued)

Unit 1 emphasizes the general ways illnesses are different. These concepts are repeated in each unit, so that in Unit 4, when AIDS is introduced, students can understand both why AIDS is a serious disease and how it is different from the diseases that commonly affect children.

Unit Summary

Activity 1. What Is Health? What Is Illness? (10 minutes): The teacher guides a *discussion* on students' experiences of health and illness. By sharing their experiences, students learn that it is normal to be sick sometimes.

Activity 2. Different Illnesses (10 minutes): Students *brainstorm* a list of illnesses they have had or have heard about. The teacher uses several *stories* to help students understand that different illnesses have different causes, different symptoms and different treatments.

Activity 3. If You're Sick, Can I Get It? (15 minutes): The teacher tells a *story* about 2 good friends, one of whom is sick, to demonstrate the differences between communicable and non-communicable illnesses.

Activity 4. Getting Help When I Am Sick (15 minutes): The class *discusses* resources students can go to when ill and identifies people to go to with questions. The teacher acknowledges that children often worry about illnesses and health. Younger children complete an *activity sheet* and older children complete a *drawing* to explore these themes.

Evaluation. How Illnesses Are Different (15–25 minutes): Younger children complete an *activity sheet* and older children complete a *drawing* to show what they have learned about differences among illnesses. The teacher guides a *discussion* about the images in the activity sheets or drawings, and emphasizes that different illnesses have different causes, symptoms and treatments.

Family Activity. The *family activity* encourages students to talk with their parents about a time they were ill, who helped them, and how they got better.

Developmental Framework

- Younger students may have less information to volunteer in the brainstorming exercise in Activity 1, so you may need to fill in this discussion.

- An activity sheet is available as an alternative to the drawing exercise in Activity 4.
- An activity sheet is available as an alternative to the drawing exercise in the Evaluation.

Terms to Use
- illness
- health
- different causes
- different symptoms
- different treatments

Review Teacher Content Summaries for Unit 1:
- **Helping Young Children Understand How Illnesses are Different** (p. 133)
- **Communicable and Non-Communicable Illnesses** (p. 135)

Get Ready *For Activity 3 have:*
- 5–10 pieces of colored yarn, each about 3 feet long
- tape or pins
- 2 large, cut-out human figures for bulletin board (You can also draw large figures on the board.)
- **Illness Picture Cards,** from Teacher Page 1.1 *(for younger students)*
- strips of paper *(for older students)* (You can also write the names of illnesses on the board.)

For Activity 4 have:
- **Getting Help When I Am Sick** (Student Activity Sheet 1.2) *(for younger students)*
- drawing materials *(for older students)*

For Evaluation have:
- crayons
- **How Illnesses Are Different** (Student Activity Sheet 1.3) *(for younger students)*
- drawing materials *(for older students)*
- **Once When I Was Sick** (Family Activity Sheet 1.4) *(for all students)*

How AIDS Works: Grades K–3

Activity 1

What Is Health? What Is Sickness?

Time	10 minutes
Objective	Students will be able to explain that feeling healthy is different from feeling sick, and that it is normal to be sick sometimes.

Introduce curriculum Tell students that today they are going to start a series of lessons about health and sickness. Knowing more about health and sickness will help them stay healthy and feel better.

Students notice physical feelings Ask students to close their eyes and pay attention to their bodies for just a moment. Ask students:

- How does your body feel?
- What is your body doing?
- Are you feeling sleepy and tired?
- Do you have lots of energy and want to move around?

Discuss health and sickness Ask students to open their eyes. Talk about how their bodies are feeling. As you gather information from them, ask the following questions:

- Does this sound like a healthy group of people?
- What makes you think this a healthy (or not a healthy) group?
- Have any of you ever been sick? When you were sick, did you feel differently from the way you feel today? How did you feel?

Make the following points:
- Feeling healthy is different from feeling sick.
- It is normal to feel sick sometimes. Everyone feels sick sometimes.

Activity 1 **What Is Health? What Is Sickness?** *continued*

Ongoing Assessment Use the following questions to assess whether students understand the difference between feeling physically healthy and feeling sick, and that feeling sick is something that happens to everyone sometimes.

- When people say they feel healthy, what does that mean?

    Feeling healthy means you have energy; you feel good; you don't feel sick.

- When people say they feel sick, what does that mean?

    Feeling sick means you don't feel good; you might have a headache or stomach ache; you feel crummy.

- How do we know it is normal to be sick sometimes?

    Everyone feels sick sometimes; feeling sick is something that happens to everyone.

Activity 2

Different Illnesses

Time	10 minutes
Objective	Students will be able to explain three ways illnesses can be different from one another: different causes, symptoms and treatments.
Teacher Background	• Helping Young Children Understand How Illnesses Are Different (p. 133).

Brainstorm list of illnesses Acknowledge that there are many different kinds of illnesses. Ask students to name some of the illnesses they have had or have heard about. Write these on the board.

Explain differences among illnesses Explain to students that there are many different kinds of illnesses, and that each illness has things about it that are different from other illnesses.

Different illnesses have different causes (different ways someone gets them), different symptoms (each illness makes people sick in different ways), and different medicines or treatments (there are different things people can do to get better).

Tell a story about illness Pick 2 of the illnesses on the list and develop a story about them that shows ways they are different (different causes, different symptoms, different treatments). The kind of difference the story illustrates is not as important as the idea that illnesses are different from each other.

Examples:

> *When Michael went on a trip to Chicago, he wasn't able to visit his cousin Jamal because Jamal had the flu, and Michael's mother was afraid Michael might get it. But when Michael came home,*

(continued)

18   Unit 1: Different Illnesses

Activity 2 Different Illnesses, *continued*

his sister Sheila had an asthma attack, and his mother let him play in the same room as Sheila. Why? Because a flu can easily be passed between two people, and asthma is not passed between people. Different illnesses have different causes—different ways someone gets them.

When Adelle had a runny nose, cough and a fever, her father told her she had a cold. A few months later, Adelle had a fever and little red spots all over her stomach, arms and legs. What do you suppose her father told her this time? Maybe he told her she had measles or chicken pox, and took her to the doctor to be sure. The way a cold makes you sick is different from the way measles make you sick. Each illness makes you sick in different ways. Different illnesses have different symptoms.

Sally took some cough medicine when she had a cough. Later in the year, when she had a headache, would she take more of the cough medicine? Why not? Because these are different illnesses, and Sally will need to do different things to get over the different illnesses. Remember, the medicine or treatment for one illness might be different from that for another. You might take medicine to get better from one illness and just rest to get better from another.

Students tell stories Ask students to pick out 2 illnesses and tell a story that shows a way the illnesses are different. You can also select 2 illnesses that are clearly different (e.g., a cold or food poisoning) and ask students to tell a story that shows a way these illnesses are different. Stories can be true or made up. Ask for volunteers to tell their stories.

Confirm and validate responses that illustrate differences in cause, symptom or treatment. Clarify and correct student impressions where necessary.

How AIDS Works: Grades K–3

Activity 2   Different Illnesses, *continued*

Ongoing Assessment   Use the following question to assess whether students understand that different illnesses have different causes, different symptoms and different treatments.

- What are some of the things that make one illness different from another?

    There are different ways to get them. Each illness makes people sick in different ways. There are different things people can do to get better from different illnesses.

Activity 3

If You're Sick, Can I Get It?

Time	15 minutes
Objective	Students will be able to identify or describe the difference between illnesses that are communicable (you can catch them from someone) and illnesses that are non-communicable (you can't catch them from someone).
Teacher Background	• Communicable and Non-Communicable Illnesses (p. 135).
Materials	• human figures • pieces of colored yarn • tape or pins • Illness Picture Cards OR strips of paper

Tell story to illustrate communicable and non-communicable illnesses

Explain to students that some illnesses can be caught from other people, and some illnesses cannot be caught. They probably already know something about this.

Draw a picture on the board of 2 people, or place 2 large cut-out figures on a bulletin board. Tell students this story:

This is a picture of Joe and Susy. They are good friends, and they spend a lot of time together.

For younger students:

Hold up each **Illness Picture Card** and ask students if they have ever heard about this illness. Ask a volunteer to briefly describe the illness.

Post the cards under the picture of Joe.

For older students:

Ask students to think about some of the different illnesses they know about. Write these on the board underneath the picture of Joe,

(continued)

Activity 3 **If You're Sick, Can I Get It?** *continued*

or write them on strips of paper and post the strips under the cut-out of Joe on the bulletin board.

Add to this list yourself if necessary, to make sure there is a selection of both communicable and non-communicable illnesses.

Students evaluate illnesses

Continue the story:

Let's imagine that Joe has been quite a sick boy lately. I wonder if Susy needs to worry about getting sick if she spends time with Joe.

Ask students to evaluate each of the illnesses on Joe's list. Example:

Joe has a cold. If Susy visits Joe, could she catch his cold?

Students should acknowledge that Susy could catch Joe's cold. Explain that this is because the cold is caused by germs, and the germs can spread from Joe to Susy from coughs, shared cups, Susy touching a tissue Joe has used and then touching her mouth, etc.

Attach a piece of colored yarn to the board so it runs from the name or picture card of the illness to the space under the picture of Susy. A student could help with this. This shows that a cold is an illness that one person can catch from another.

Repeat for the other listed illnesses.

Example:

And now Joe has poison ivy. If Susy visits Joe, could she catch his poison ivy?

Poison ivy cannot be passed from person to person, so no yarn is placed under the pictures.

Discuss ways to prevent illness

When all the illnesses on the list have been discussed, explain that many illnesses can be prevented. If people know how a disease is passed from person to person, they can often figure out how to keep from getting it.

Review the list of illnesses again, and discuss ways to prevent the communicable ones. Remove the pieces of yarn once the prevention strategies for an illness have been discussed.

(continued)

Activity 3   **If You're Sick, Can I Get It?** *continued*

Make the point that people can take simple steps to protect themselves from many illnesses, even those that are passed from person to person.

Reassure students Before closing this activity, reassure students that though there are many germs in their environment, the body has a lot of clever ways to protect itself. Later, (in Unit 3), this will be discussed in more detail. For now, it is important for children to understand that their bodies are working all the time to keep them safe and healthy. By taking some of the steps talked about today (washing hands, having others cover their mouths when coughing), they can help their bodies protect them.

Ongoing Assessment Use the following question to assess whether students can distinguish between communicable and non-communicable diseases.

■ What makes an illness like asthma or poison ivy different from an illness like a cold or chicken pox? (Prompt: Do you need to worry about catching poison ivy or asthma?)

You can catch a cold or chicken pox from someone, but you can't catch asthma.

How AIDS Works: Grades K–3

Activity 4

Getting Help When I Am Sick

Time	15 minutes
Objective	Students will be able to list appropriate steps to take in response to signs or symptoms of illness or questions about illness.
Materials	• Getting Help When I Am Sick (1.2) OR drawing materials

Identify people who can help when students are sick

Ask students to think about a time they did not feel well. Did they talk to anyone or get any help when they were sick?

In this discussion, make the point that there are people children and adults can go to for help when they are sick. Examples:

- parents
- doctor
- school nurse
- teacher
- other relatives
- friends
- friends' parents

Ask students: *What kind of help did these people offer?*

In this discussion, emphasize that there are steps people can take to get better when they are sick. Examples:

- "My mother told me to go to bed"—getting rest.
- "My brother took me to the clinic"—seeking medical care.
- "My grandma took my temperature"—gathering information.

Activity 4   **Getting Help When I Am Sick,** *continued*

Acknowledge worry about illness

Acknowledge that many children often worry about illnesses. They might worry about whether they are sick, or whether they have a serious illness. They might worry about a friend, or someone in their family. Ask students if they can think of a time they had a question about health or illness. Did they talk to anyone about their question?

In this discussion, make the point that many of the same people children can go to when they are sick are also people to turn to with questions about health or sickness (e.g., parents, doctor, school nurse, teacher, other relatives, friends' parents).

Students complete assignment

For younger students:

Distribute Student Activity Sheet 1.2, **Getting Help When I Am Sick**. Have students complete it by circling the pictures that show ways they have gotten help when they were sick.

1. Told an adult they were sick.
2. Had their temperature taken.
3. Received medicine.
4. Stayed home in bed.

For older students:

Have students draw a picture about a time they did not feel well and someone helped them in some way. Students with writing skills can also write a story about the picture.

Ongoing Assessment

Use the following questions to assess whether students understand appropriate steps to take in response to signs of illness or when they have questions about illness.

- If you were feeling sick, whom could you talk to?

    Parents, doctor, school nurse, teacher, other relatives, friends, friends' parents.

- Imagine you had a question about an illness. Maybe you wondered if you were getting sick, or had questions about an illness a friend has. Whom could you go to with your question?

    Parents, doctor, school nurse, teacher, other relatives, friends' parents.

Evaluation

How Illnesses Are Different

Time	15–25 minutes
Objective	Students will be able to describe the general ways illnesses are different, including that they have different causes, symptoms and treatments.
Materials	• crayons • How Illnesses Are Different (1.3) OR drawing materials • Once When I Was Sick (1.4)

■ **Note:** For older students, this activity can be done in 2 segments. In the first, the students draw their pictures. In the second, the pictures are posted around the room and the teacher facilitates a discussion.

Review differences about illness

Ask students to remember the 3 differences about illness they have discussed:

- Different illnesses have different causes—different ways someone gets them.
- They have different symptoms—each illness makes people feel sick in different ways.
- They have different treatments—there are different things people can do to get better from different illnesses.

Students complete assignment

For younger students:

Distribute Student Activity Sheet 1.3, **How Illnesses Are Different**. Explain that the activity sheet shows 2 children, each with a different illness. The boy has the flu. The girl has poison ivy (or poison oak, depending on which region of the country you live in).

Ask students to describe what they see in the pictures. Look for and confirm answers that refer to different causes, different symptoms and different treatments.

(continued)

Unit 1: Different Illnesses

Evaluation   **How Illnesses Are Different,** *continued*

Ask students to describe a difference in one of these 3 areas. Ask them to circle the image that shows that kind of difference in a particular color crayon. For example, the pictures that show causes could be circled in red, those showing symptoms could be circled in blue, and those showing treatments could be circled in green.

Example:

> *One of the pictures shows the girl scratching a rash, and the boy in bed with a fever. These are symptoms—the ways illnesses make people feel sick. Use a blue crayon to circle the pictures that show different ways different illnesses can make people feel sick.*

Use the final panels, where both children are well, to emphasize that the illnesses children usually get are not serious. They are usually easy to treat and the child feels better soon.

For older students:

Write the words *Causes, Symptoms* and *Treatments* on the board.

Distribute drawing materials. Ask students to draw a picture showing a way illnesses can be different. Students with writing skills can also write a short paragraph about the drawing.

Ask students to decide what their drawing shows most: different causes, different symptoms or different treatments. If it shows different causes, have them put a "C" somewhere on the paper and draw a circle around it. If the drawing shows different symptoms, ask them to put an "S," if different treatments, a "T."

Identify 3 places in the classroom for students to post their pictures. One will be for pictures that show different causes; one for those that show symptoms, and one for those that show treatments. Have students post their drawings in the appropriate area.

When this is completed, have students move about the room to look at the different pictures. Ask them to think about the areas of difference shown in the drawings.

After students return to their seats, facilitate a discussion that reviews the differences among illnesses. Fill in any important points that might be missing from the group of pictures.

(continued)

Evaluation   **How Illnesses Are Different,** *continued*

> ■ **Note:** The discussion might also look at which category has the most drawings, which has the least, and ask students why they think this is the case. This will give you an opportunity to learn more about what students understand about differences among illnesses.

Summarize   Summarize the important areas of learning in Unit 1. Cover the following points:

- Different illnesses have different causes, symptoms and treatments.
- There are some illnesses one person can catch from another and some that one person cannot catch from another.
- It is normal to be sick sometimes. Everyone gets sick sometimes.
- There are people students can go to for help if they feel sick, or for answers if they have questions about illnesses.

Family Activity   Ask students to take their activity sheets or drawings from this unit home to share with their parents. Distribute Family Activity Sheet 1.4, **Once When I Was Sick,** and ask students to complete the sheet with their parents.

TEACHER PAGE 1.1

Illness Picture Cards

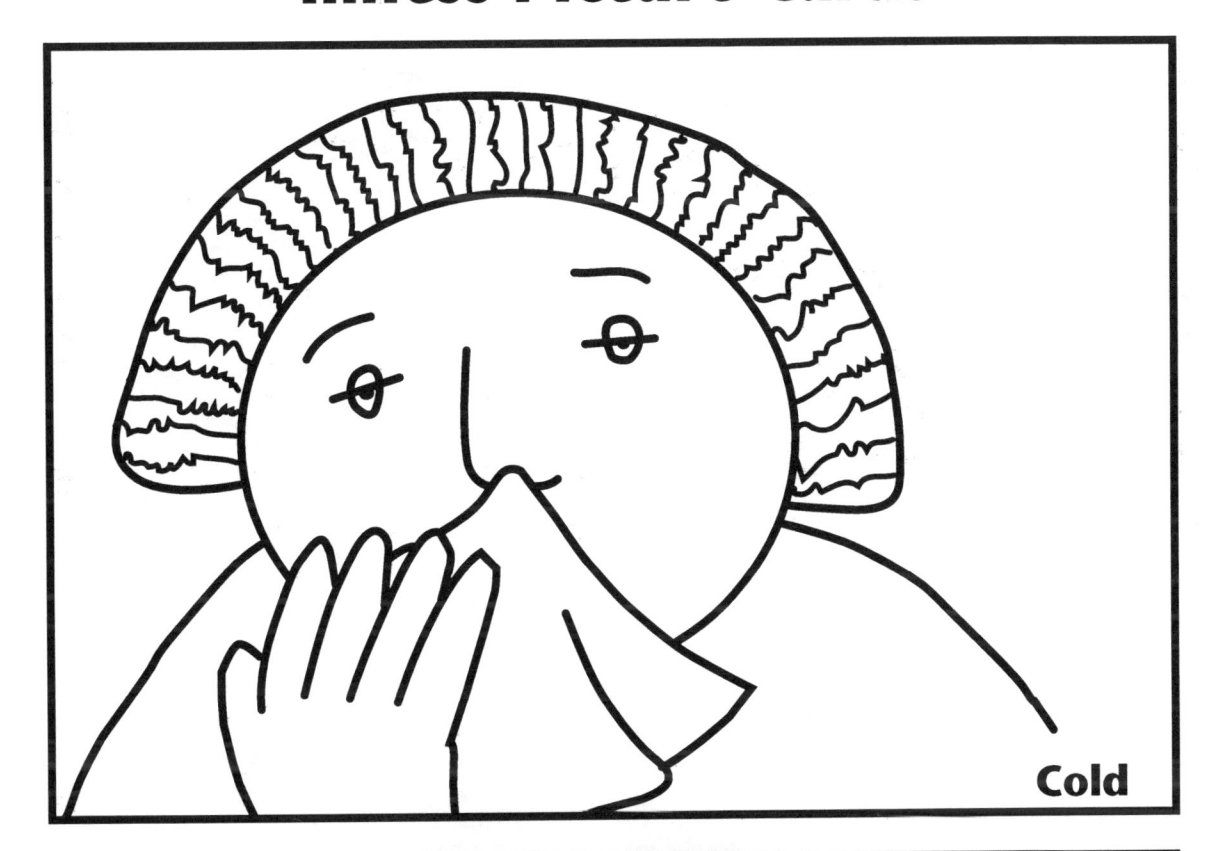

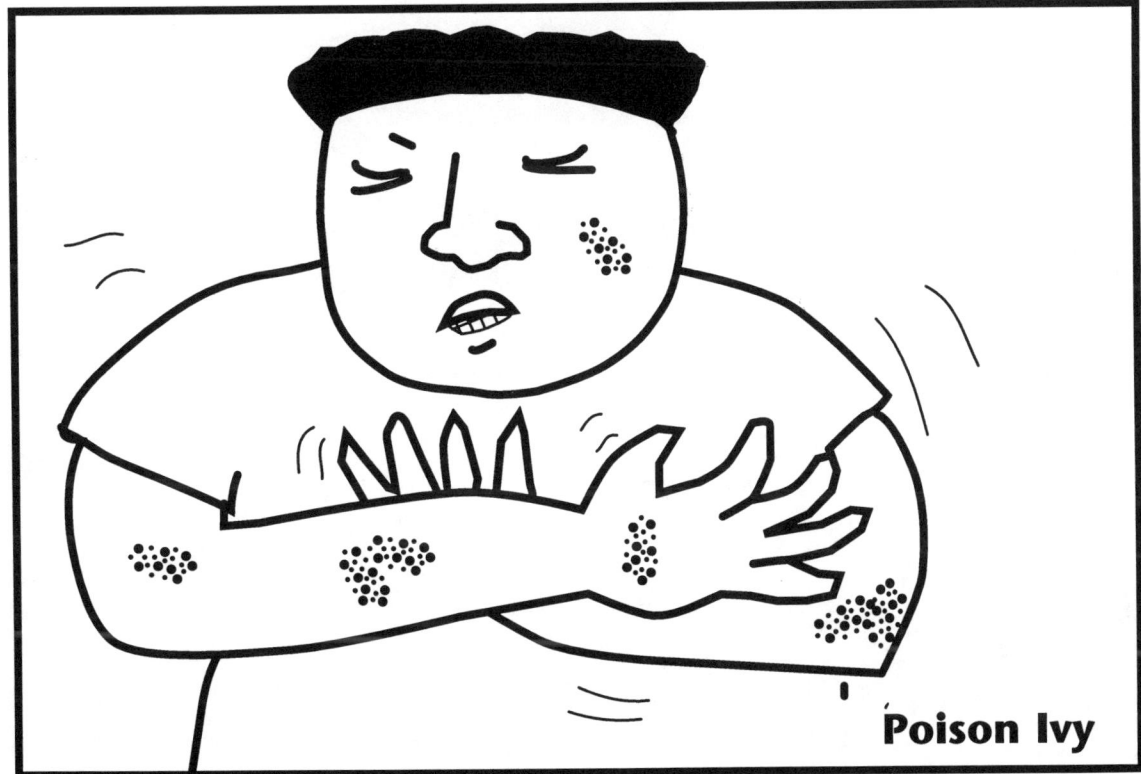

Cold

Poison Ivy

© ETR Associates

How AIDS Works: Grades K–3

29

TEACHER PAGE 1.1
continued

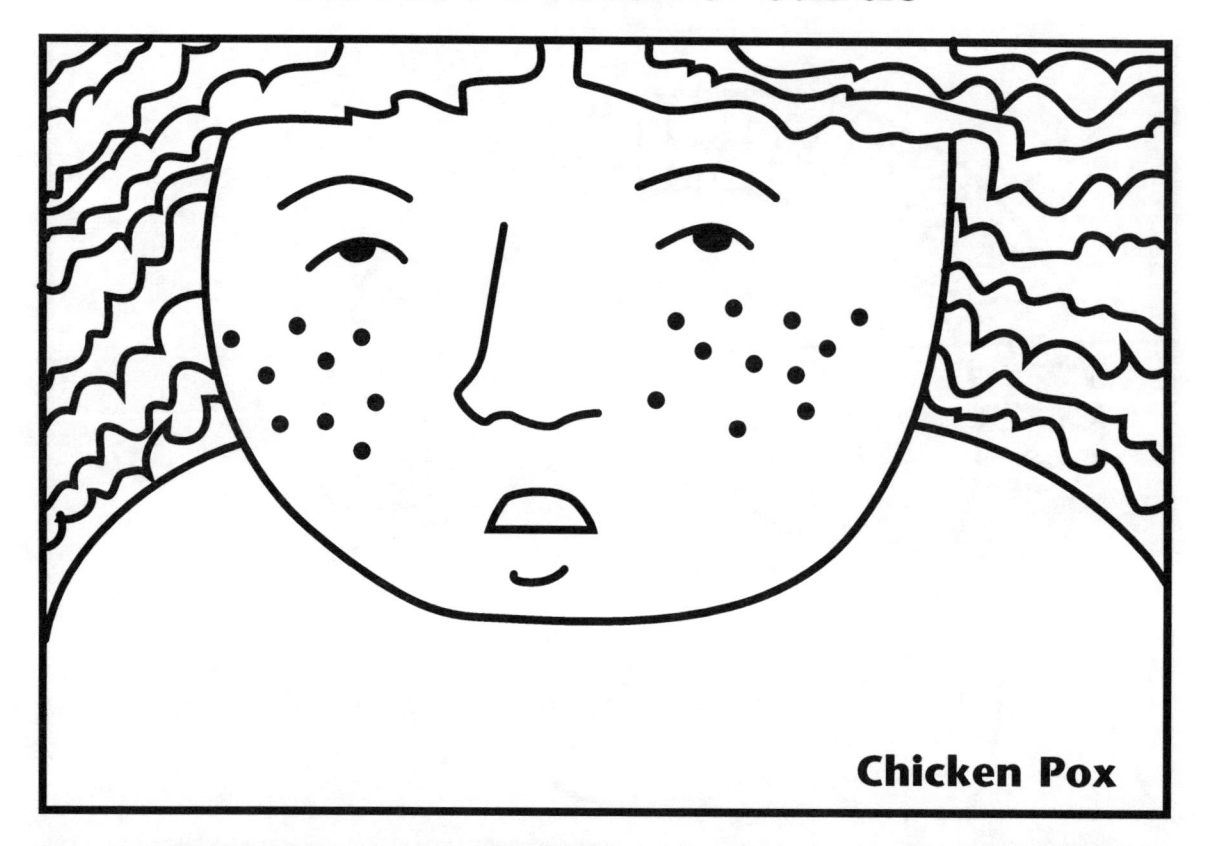

Illness Picture Cards

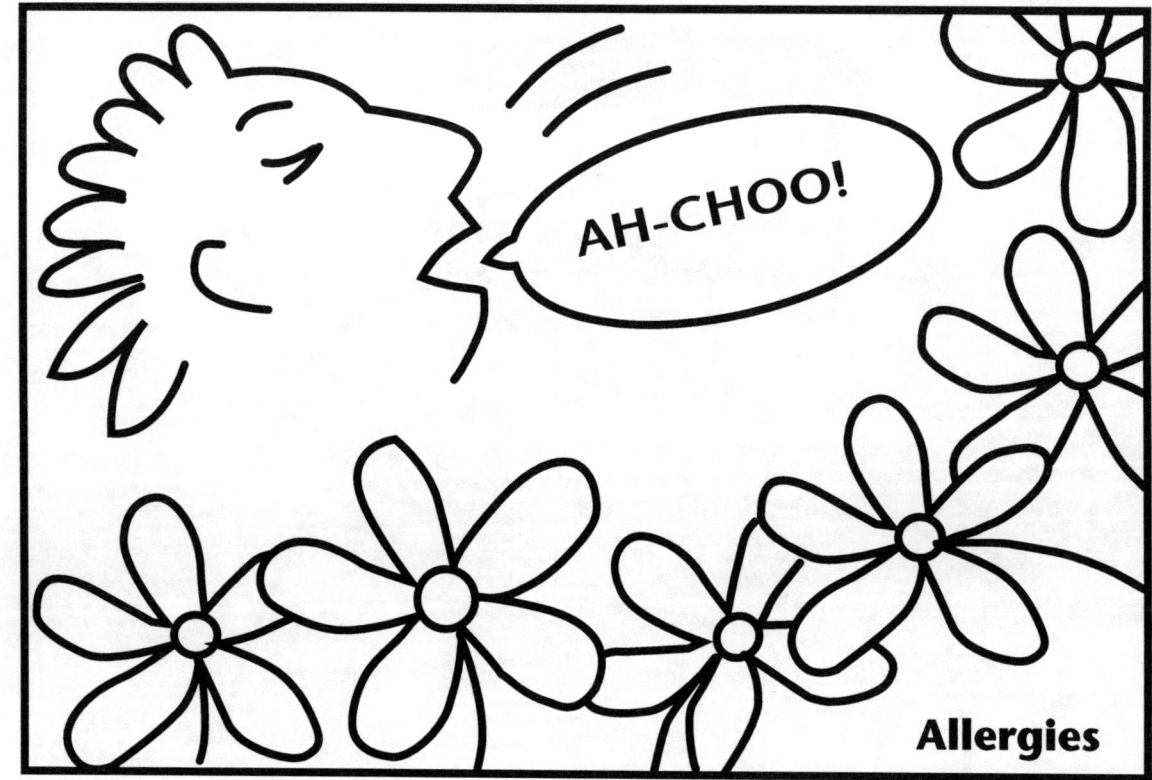

Chicken Pox

AH-CHOO!

Allergies

30

Unit 1: Different Illnesses

TEACHER PAGE 1.1
continued

Illness Picture Cards

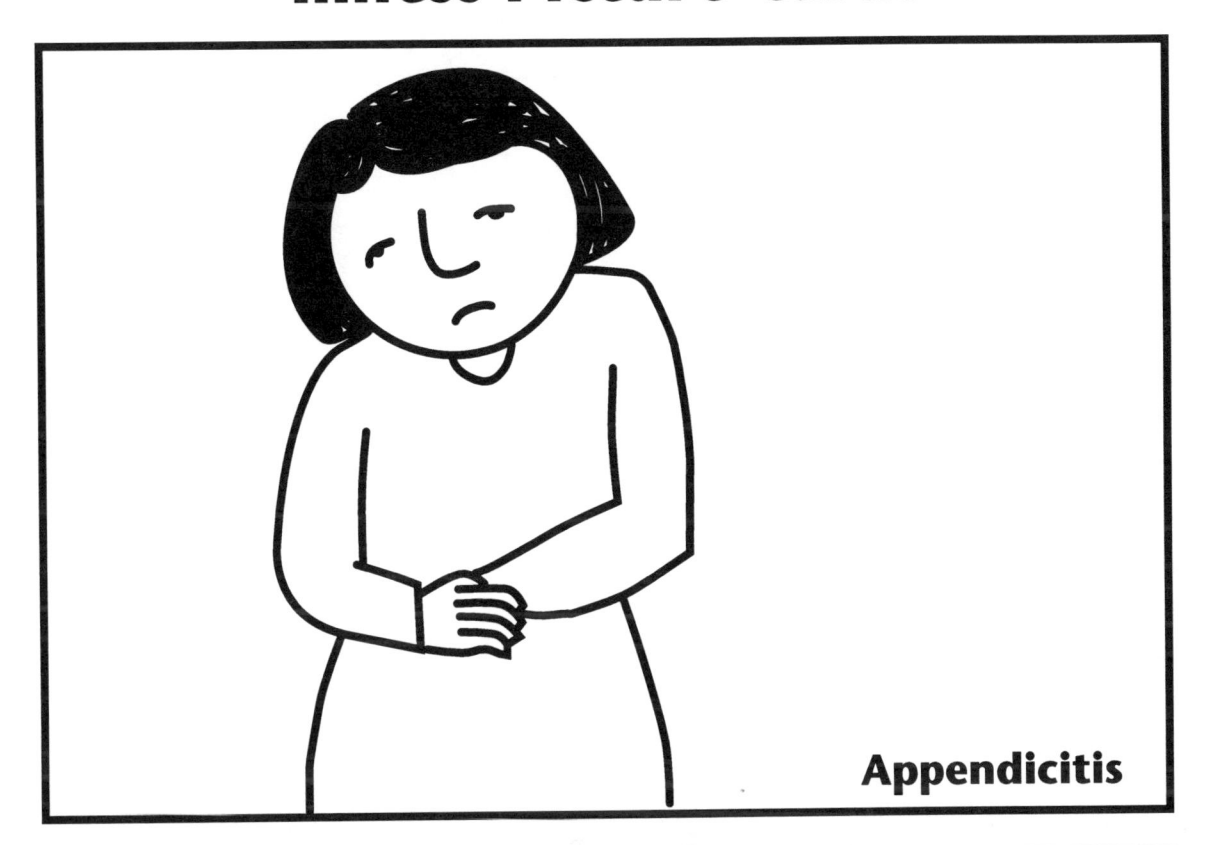

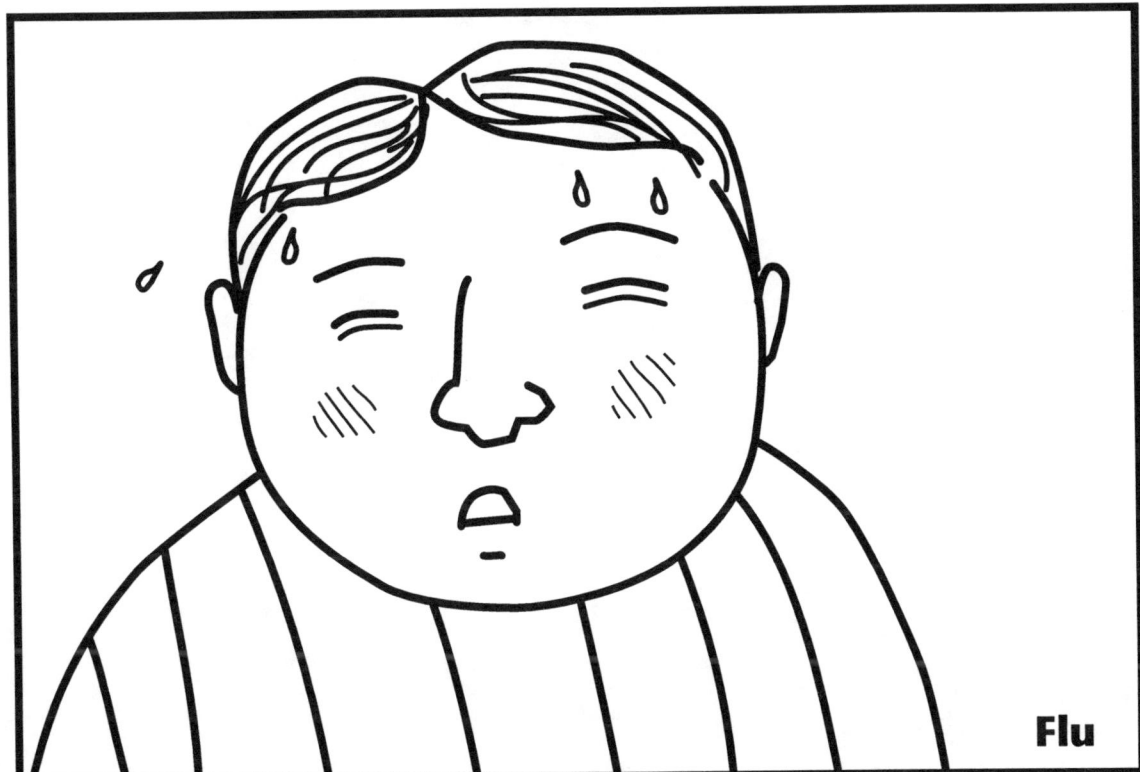

Appendicitis

Flu

How AIDS Works: Grades K–3

STUDENT ACTIVITY SHEET 1.2

Name _____

Getting Help When I Am Sick

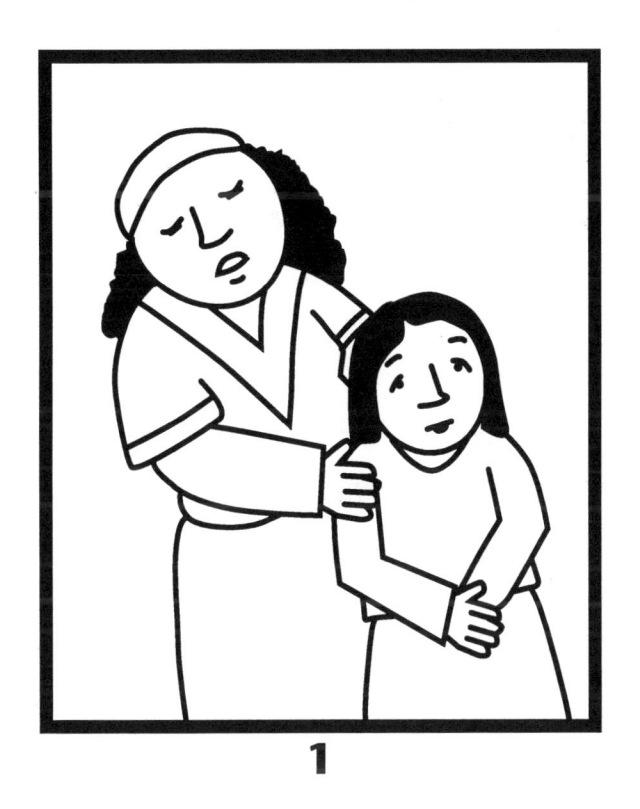

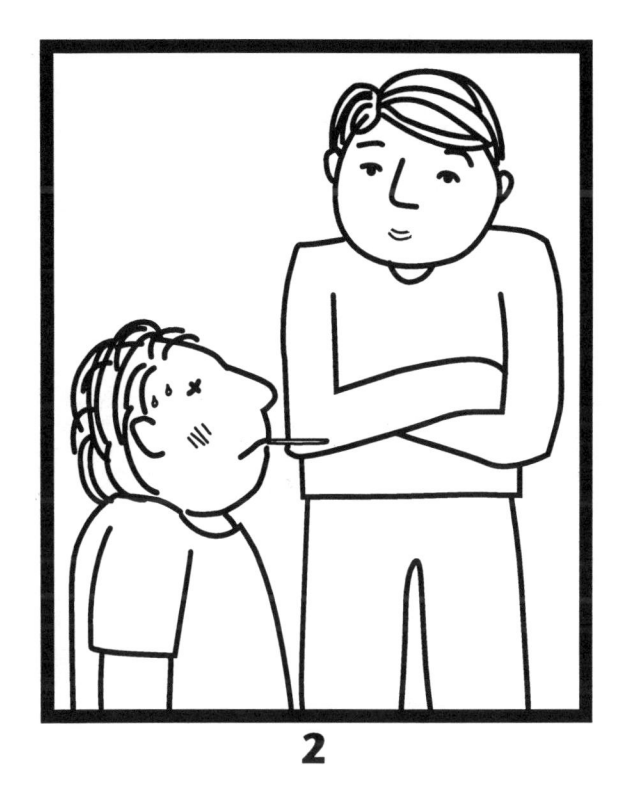

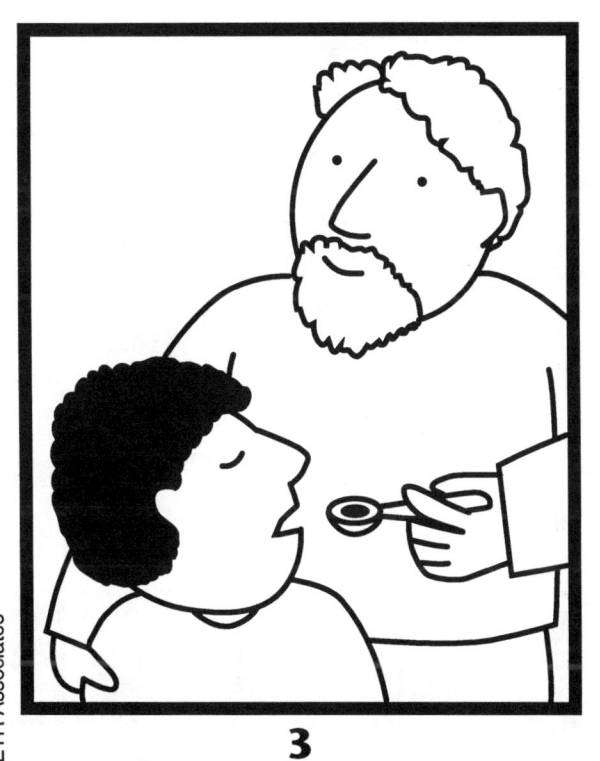

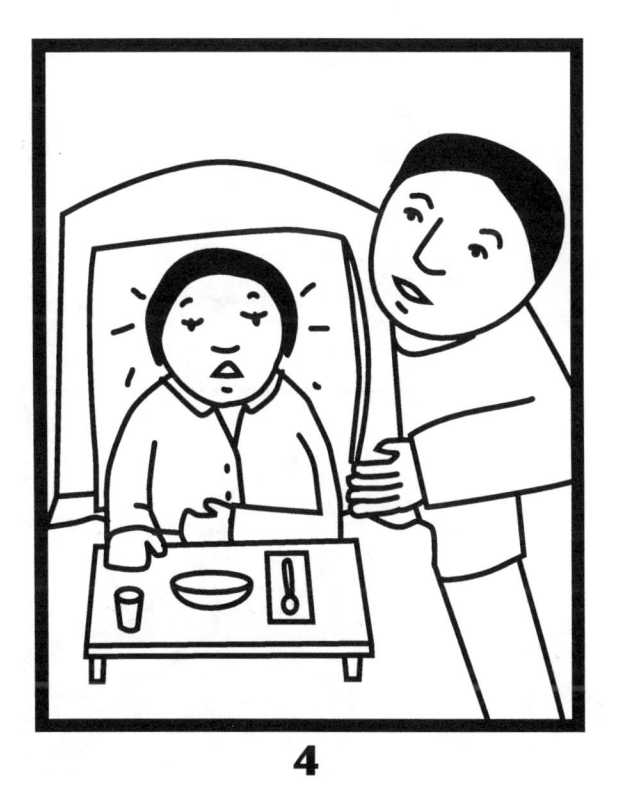

1

2

3

4

How AIDS Works: Grades K–3

33

STUDENT ACTIVITY SHEET 1.3

Name _____

How Illnesses Are Different

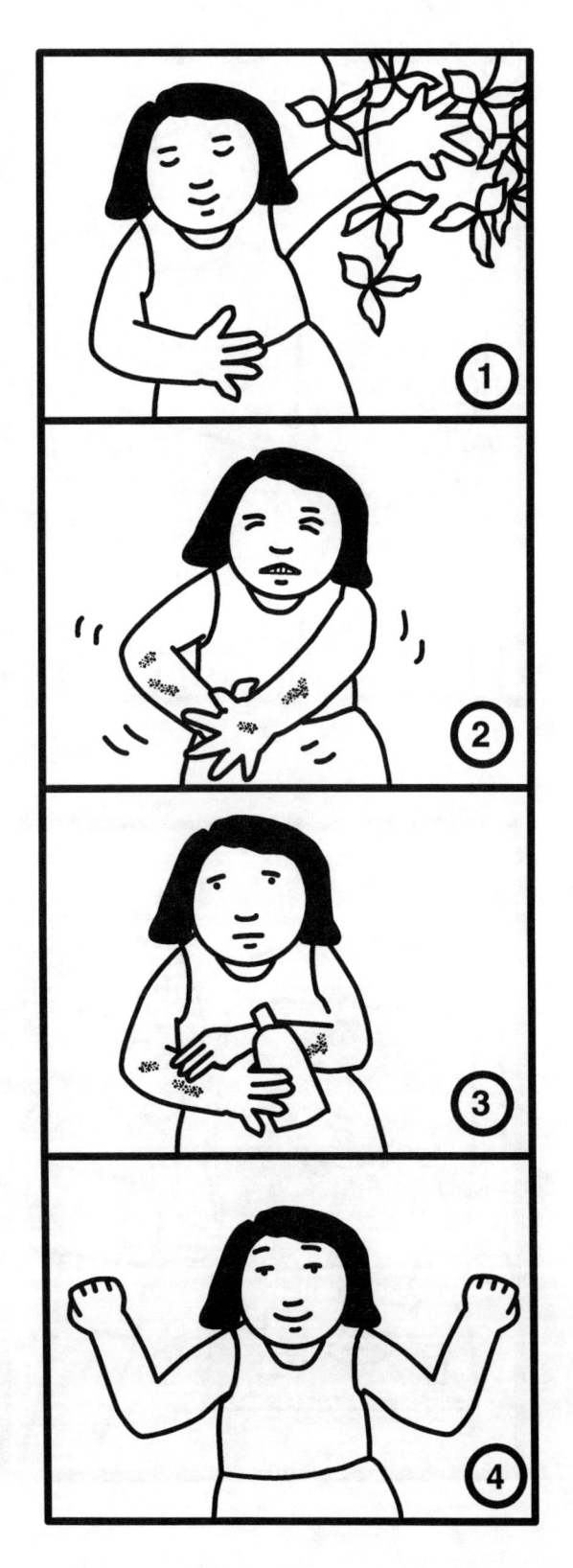

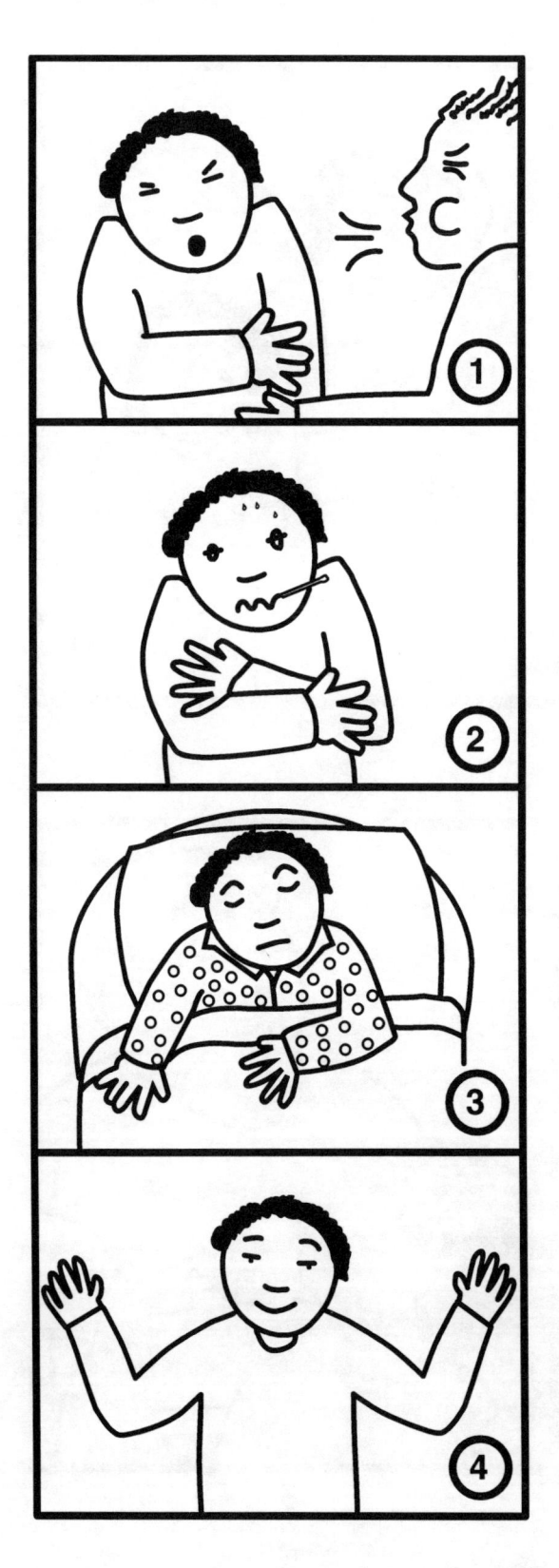

Unit 1: Different Illnesses

FAMILY ACTIVITY SHEET 1.4

Once When I Was Sick

Dear Parents,

Your child's class is now participating in a 6-unit curriculum on AIDS. In Unit 1, students are learning the general ways illnesses can differ: there are different ways someone gets them, different symptoms, and different ways to treat different illnesses.

These are the concepts for Unit 1:

1. It is normal to be sick sometimes. Everyone gets sick sometimes.

2. Different illnesses have different causes (different ways someone gets them), different symptoms (each illness makes people feel sick in different ways) and different treatments (there are different things people can do to get better from different illnesses).

3. There are some illnesses one person can catch from another (communicable), and some illnesses one person cannot catch from another (non-communicable).

Student Work

As part of these lessons, students completed an activity sheet or a drawing about a time they did not feel well and someone helped them in some way. Please ask your child to show you the activity sheet or drawing. Then discuss the following questions:

1. What were some of the ways you were feeling sick? (Ask your child to list 3.)

2. What are some things you can do to take care of yourself if you start to feel sick? (Ask your child to list 3.)

If you can think of a time when you became ill and were helped by someone else, you could tell your child about your experience.

© ETR Associates

(continued)

How AIDS Works: Grades K–3

FAMILY ACTIVITY SHEET 1.4
continued

Further Information

The first 3 units of the curriculum teach about illnesses in general. Beginning in Unit 4, students will be learning specifically about AIDS.

You will not need to have all the facts about AIDS to talk about the topic with your child and respond to questions. If you would like further information about the lessons, please feel free to call me at _____.

If you have questions about AIDS, you can call the National AIDS Hotline at 1-800-342-AIDS, or the local AIDS Hotline at _____.
If your child asks you something about AIDS and you do not know the answer, you could call the hotline together for more information.

Sincerely,

_____
(Teacher name)

Unit 2

Different Ways to Be Sick

Time 55 minutes

Unit Objective Students will be able to describe some of the differences between illnesses and understand that most illnesses children get are not serious.

Concepts
1. Some germs can live in many different places—the air, the surface of a desk, hands, in the body. Other germs can only live in a few places—inside the body, for example.
2. Some communicable illnesses are easy to pass between people. Some are hard to pass.
3. Some illnesses are very serious and hard to treat. Others are not so serious, and are easy to treat. Most get better on their own.
4. Most of the illnesses children get are not serious, and are easy to treat.

Overview Young children often have mistaken concepts about germs that can lead to confusion. For example, they may think there is only one kind of germ, that one germ can cause all illnesses, or that all illness, including AIDS, can be caused by germs commonly found in children's day-to-day environment—on desks, doorknobs or eating utensils. It is understandable that children with these misconceptions would be concerned about their own susceptibility to AIDS.

Unit 2 helps students add sophistication to the knowledge they already have about germs. The emphasis is on helping students learn

(continued)

the difference between their common experiences with illness and some of the special circumstances that apply to more serious illnesses. This includes understanding that different germs cause different illnesses; that different germs live and grow in different kinds of environments; and that, while illnesses they commonly see are usually easy to pass to other people, other illnesses are hard to pass. This is an essential concept to have in place if children are to understand how AIDS is different from other illnesses.

Unit 2 responds to children's anxieties about AIDS and other serious illnesses by explaining the difference between serious, hard-to-treat illnesses and benign, easy-to-treat illnesses, and provides the reassurance that most of the illnesses children get are not serious.

Unit Summary

Activity 1. What Is A Germ? (15 minutes): After a brief *review* of concepts in Unit 1, the teacher presents a short *lecture* about germs, including what they are, where they can be found and how they are spread from person to person. In a *demonstration,* students cough into their hands and feel the moisture left by the tiny drops of saliva that carry germs.

Activity 2. Seeing Is Believing: Watching "Germs" Pass (15 minutes): In a *demonstration* and *interactive exercise,* students who have oil and glitter on their hands shake hands with other students and pass the glitter—representing germs—to them. In *discussion,* the teacher emphasizes that some kinds of germs can live in many different places, but others can live in only a few places. General prevention strategies are also discussed.

Activity 3. Serious and Not-So-Serious Illnesses (10 minutes): In a *lecture,* the teacher explains that some diseases are serious and some are not, and the differences between them. The point is made that most of the illnesses children get are not serious, and get better on their own or are easy to treat. Optional *discussion questions* are included to address students' feelings, concerns and anxieties if a classmate or other person they know has a serious illness.

Evaluation. Elizabeth and Mrs. Shaw: A Story (15 minutes): A *story* helps assess students' understanding of the differences between serious and not-so-serious illnesses.

Family Activity. The *family activity* encourages students to talk with their parents about the differences between serious and not-so-serious illnesses.

Developmental Framework
- Throughout the discussion activities, younger students may have less information to volunteer, so you may need to fill in the discussion.

Terms to Use
- germ
- easy-to-pass illness
- hard-to-pass illness
- serious illness
- not-so-serious illness

Review Teacher Content Summaries for Unit 2:
- **Germs and Germ Theory** (p. 142)
- **Discussing Serious Illness with Young Children** (p. 143)

Get Ready *For Activity 2 have:*
- vegetable oil
- glitter or nutmeg (*Note:* glitter sticks or pastes can also be used.)
- hand soap
- sink with running water or bowl of warm, soapy water
- paper towels, several for each student

For Evaluation have:
- crayons
- **Elizabeth and Mrs. Shaw: A Story** (Teacher Page 2.1)
- **Elizabeth and Mrs. Shaw** (Student Activity Sheet 2.2) *(for younger students)*
- drawing materials *(for older students)*
- **Different Ways to Be Sick** (Family Activity Sheet 2.3) *(for all students)*

Activity 1

What Is a Germ?

Time	15 minutes
Objective	Students will be able to identify a germ and describe two ways germs can be passed from person to person.
Teacher Background	• Germs and Germ Theory (p. 142)

Review concepts Use the Review Guide (p. 157) to review concepts from Unit 1. Areas where students have demonstrated successful understanding of the concepts can be reviewed briefly; review those where concepts may still present a challenge in more depth.

Ask one or more of the questions provided, confirming answers that demonstrate understanding of the concepts and clarifying any misconceptions.

Introduce activity Remind students that in Unit 1, they discussed the story of Susy and Joe. The class talked about germs, and some of the ways germs can cause illness. Today, they are going to learn more about germs: what they are, what they do, and steps people can take to avoid germs and keep from getting sick.

Describe germs Describe germs (or, for older students, ask, "What is a germ?").

- A germ is a special kind of living thing so small people cannot see it.
- There are many different kinds of germs. Some germs can cause sickness if they get inside a person's body.

Explain where germs can be found (or, for older students, ask, "Where can germs be found?").

(continued)

Activity 1   What Is a Germ? *continued*

- Germs can be found in our hair, on our hands, on a pencil. There are germs almost everywhere.

Describe how germs can be spread (or, for older students, ask, "How are germs spread?").

- Touching things that have germs on them
- Using objects, like cups or forks or tissues, that have been used by someone else
- Coughing and sneezing
- Blood-to-blood contact

Demonstrate one way germs can spread

Ask students to feel the palm of one hand with the fingers of the other. Are their hands dry or moist?

Have students place one hand close to the mouth and cough into the palm. Then ask them to feel the palm again. Are their hands dry or moist?

Most students will be able to feel more moistness on the palm of the hand after coughing. Explain that this moistness comes from small drops of saliva that enter the air when someone coughs. Often, people cannot even see these drops.

When someone has a cold, germs from their coughs can get into the air, carried in the tiny drops of saliva. Someone near the person with the cold might breathe these germs in, and then also get the cold.

Remind students to cover their mouths when coughing or sneezing, and to wash their hands after they cough or sneeze, especially if they have been sick. These steps can help protect other people from getting sick.

Discuss how to avoid germs

Inform students that people can take steps to avoid contact with germs (or, for older students, ask, "What are some ways people can avoid contact with germs?").

- Wash hands before meals, after playing outside, after coughing or sneezing, after touching something that might have germs.

(continued)

How AIDS Works: Grades K–3

Activity 1   **What Is a Germ?** *continued*

- Do not touch things that are likely to have lots of disease-causing germs on them, such as used drug needles, dead animals, animal droppings, things in trash cans, or other people's blood.
- Cover mouth when coughing or sneezing, and wash hands afterwards, so as not to spread germs to someone else.

Ongoing Assessment   Use the following questions to assess whether students understand ways germs can be spread and ways to prevent germs from being spread.

■ What are some of the ways germs can be passed from one person to another?

Touching things that have germs on them; using objects, such as cups, forks or tissues, that have been used by someone else; coughing and sneezing; touching blood; blood-to-blood contact.

■ What kinds of steps can people take to keep from passing germs?

Wash hands. Do not touch things likely to have germs on them. Cover mouth when coughing or sneezing and wash hands afterwards.

Activity 2

Seeing Is Believing: Watching "Germs" Pass

Time	15 minutes
Objective	Students will be able to explain that some germs live in many places and can be passed easily from person to person, while others live in only a few places and are harder to pass.
Materials	• vegetable oil • glitter or nutmeg • hand soap • water • paper towels

Introduce activity

Explain to students that, while it is impossible to see germs with your eyes, it is easy to see one way germs could be spread from person to person.

Demonstrate how germs are passed

Have one-third of the students participate in this first step. Put a little vegetable oil into students' palms (about a quarter teaspoon each) and ask them to rub their palms together. Then sprinkle a little glitter (or nutmeg) onto students' palms and ask them to rub their palms together again.

Warn students not to touch their clothing while they have oil on their hands, because it will stain.

Tell the students to think of the glitter as germs, and ask them to watch what happens next.

Have each of these students shake hands with one other student who does not have oil on his or her hands. The second set of students will find that the oil and glitter transfers to their hands.

Have the second set of students shake hands with the rest of the students who have no oil on their hands. Most of these students will also find that the oil and glitter transfers.

How AIDS Works: Grades K–3

Activity 2   Seeing Is Believing, *continued*

Discuss the demonstration Ask students to describe what happened. Help them make the connection between the glitter passing from person to person, which they can see, and germs passing from person to person, which they cannot see.

Explain that washing hands with soap and water can remove germs, and will also remove the oil and glitter.

Have students wash their hands thoroughly to remove all of the oil.

Explain role of skin Explain briefly that the skin plays an important role in protecting the body from germs. Healthy skin helps keep germs outside the body, where they cannot cause sickness. Regular washing of hands helps keep skin healthy.

Clarify different types of germs Make the point that real germs that pass from person to person the easy way these "glitter germs" do can live in many different places.

Explain that other kinds of germs can live in only a few places—inside the body, for example, or in the blood. These other kinds of germs do *not* pass easily from person to person. They do not live on hands, desktops, doorknobs or cups, so people do not come into contact with these other kinds of germs in usual, day-to-day activities.

Reassure students Before closing this activity, once again reassure students that their bodies are working all the time to keep them safe from disease. By taking some simple steps such as washing their hands, they can give their bodies some help in that task.

Ongoing Assessment Use the following questions to assess whether students understand that some kinds of germs live in many places and can be passed easily from person to person, while others live in only a few places and are more difficult to pass.

■ What did you learn about how germs pass from person to person?

Some germs can pass easily; can be in lots of places; you just need to touch someone or something to get these germs on you.

(continued)

Activity 2 Seeing Is Believing, *continued*

- Not all germs pass in the easy way these "glitter germs" do. How are these other germs different?

  Other germs are harder to pass; live in only a few places; might live inside the body.

Activity 3

Serious and Not-So-Serious Illnesses

Time	10 minutes
Objective	Students will be able to describe the differences between serious and not-so-serious illnesses.
Teacher Background	• Discussing Serious Illness with Young Children (p. 143)

Review illnesses and germs

Review some of the differences the class has discussed concerning illnesses and germs:

- Different illnesses have different causes (different ways someone gets them), different symptoms (each illness makes people sick in different ways), and different treatments (there are different things people can do to get better from different illnesses).

- There are some illnesses one person can catch from another (communicable), and some illnesses that one person cannot catch from another (non-communicable).

- Some communicable illnesses are easy to pass between people. Some are hard to pass.

- Some kinds of germs can live in many different places—the air, the surface of a desk, hands, in the body. Other kinds of germs can only live in a few places—in special fluids inside the body, for example.

Let the class know that now you will be discussing another important kind of difference: that some illnesses are serious, and some illnesses are not-so-serious.

Discuss serious illness

Ask the class what kinds of things they think might happen when someone has a serious illness.

(continued)

Activity 3 Serious and Not-So-Serious Illnesses, *continued*

Look for and confirm appropriate answers, such as:
- Be very sick and feel very bad.
- Be sick for a very long time.
- Get sick over and over again.
- Go to the hospital.
- Have things go wrong with the body that do not get better.
- Not be able to work or go to school.
- Die.
- Have no treatments—no medicines or other things doctors can do to make the person get better.
- Doctors do not know whether the person will get better or not.

For students who read, you might want to make a list on the board.

Discuss not-so-serious illness Ask the class what kinds of things they think might happen when someone has a not-so-serious illness.

Look for and confirm appropriate answers, such as:
- Not feel very sick.
- Feel very sick, but not for a long time.
- Have treatments—medicines or other things doctors can do to make the person get better.
- Get better soon.
- Get better just by resting and staying at home for a few days.
- Doctors know the person will get better.

For students who read, you might want to make a list on the board.

If students have volunteered answers about serious illnesses that would better belong with the answers about not-so-serious illnesses, help them understand why you would put their answer with the "not-so-serious" list.

(continued)

How AIDS Works: Grades K–3 **47**

Activity 3   **Serious and Not-So-Serious Illnesses,** *continued*

Example:

Jana, you said you felt like you were seriously ill when you had the stomach flu because you threw up all night long. Did you have to go to the hospital? No? But you did feel really bad. Well, sometimes illnesses that are not really serious can still make us feel very sick. What makes an illness serious is not just how bad it makes a person feel. It also has to do with whether or not the person will be able to get better again, or how much doctors have to do to help the person get better. So while your flu made you feel very bad, it was not really a serious illness.

Let students know that most illnesses are not serious and people do get better from them. The illnesses children get usually are not serious.

Ongoing Assessment

Use the following question to assess whether students understand the distinction between serious and not-so-serious illnesses.

■ What are some of the differences between serious and not-so-serious illnesses?

Serious illnesses might last for a long time. There might be no medicines to make them better. The person may have to go to the hospital; might get sick over and over again; may not get better; may not be able to work or go to school; may even die.

Less serious illnesses might not make a person feel very sick or be sick for long. There are medicines or other things doctors can do to make the person better. The person may get better just by resting and staying at home for a few days. The doctor knows the person will get better.

Evaluation

Elizabeth and Mrs. Shaw: A Story

Time	15 minutes
Objective	Students will be able to describe the differences between serious and not-so-serious illnesses, and understand that most illnesses children get are not serious.
Materials	• Elizabeth and Mrs. Shaw: A Story (2.1) • crayons • Elizabeth and Mrs. Shaw (2.2) OR drawing materials • Different Ways to Be Sick (2.3)

Read story to students Read **Elizabeth and Mrs. Shaw: A Story** from Teacher Page 2.1. Show the illustration on Student Activity Sheet 2.2 as you're reading the story.

Discuss story Lead a general discussion of the story, asking some or all of the following questions:

- Elizabeth was confused about a few things at the beginning of the story. What was she confused about?

    She thought her medicine could help Mrs. Shaw get better. She worried that she might get as sick as Mrs. Shaw.

- Do you think children worry when they are around someone with a serious illness? What kinds of things do they worry about?

    Look for answers that express students' true feelings about this question. Some students may feel there is nothing to worry about, others may feel there is. There are no right or wrong answers.

- What helped Elizabeth feel better?

    She talked with Mr. Shaw and he helped her understand more about the differences between her strep throat and Mrs. Shaw's illness.

How AIDS Works: Grades K–3

| Evaluation | Elizabeth and Mrs. Shaw: A Story, *continued* |

Students respond to story

For younger students:

Distribute Student Activity Sheet 2.2, **Elizabeth and Mrs. Shaw**. Ask students to look at the picture and think about the story.

Remind students that in this story they heard about Elizabeth, who has strep throat. They also heard about Mrs. Shaw, who has cancer. One of these illnesses is serious and one is not so serious.

Ask students to circle the person who has the nonserious illness in red, and to circle the person who has the serious illness in blue.

For older students:

Distribute drawing materials. Ask students to draw a picture illustrating some part of the story. Students with writing skills can write a short paragraph about their drawing.

Optional: Students' pictures can be posted around the room for the discussion.

Review assignment and story

Guide students through a more specific discussion about the story, referring to the illustrations or their drawings as appropriate. Ask the following questions:

- In this story, we hear about Elizabeth who has strep throat. We also hear about Mrs. Shaw who has cancer. Which of these illnesses is a serious illness?
  Cancer.

- What are some of the differences between these illnesses that help us understand that Mrs. Shaw's illness is more serious than Elizabeth's?

  - *Length of illness: Elizabeth has been sick only a few days, while Mrs. Shaw has been sick for several months.*

  - *Treatments: Elizabeth's medicines work easily and well, and will help her feel better in a few days. Mrs. Shaw's medicines do not work as easily. They have not helped her feel better yet, even though she has taken them for a long time.*

  - *Length of treatment: Elizabeth will only have to take her medicines for a short time—a few days. Mrs. Shaw has to continue taking medicines for a long time—many months.*

(continued)

Evaluation Elizabeth and Mrs. Shaw: A Story, *continued*

- *Feeling better: Elizabeth's doctor and mother know she will feel better in a few days. Mrs. Shaw's doctor does not know when she will feel better.*
- *Outcome: Students may also mention outcome. Sometimes people die of cancer, but people do not die of strep throat.*

• In this story, Elizabeth, who has a not-so-serious illness, is inside, bundled up in her blanket. She cannot go outside to play. Mrs. Shaw, who has a serious illness, is walking outside. What do you think about that?

Use this part of the discussion to explain that we cannot always tell just by looking at someone whether he or she has a serious illness, and that sometimes a person with a not-so-serious illness has to rest more for a few days than someone with a serious illness.

(Optional) Talk about someone who has a serious illness

Take time here to discuss students' feelings or questions if a classmate or other member of the school community has been seriously ill. The nature of this discussion will depend on the students' actual experiences, including whether the person is now well, still seriously ill, or perhaps has died; and whether this is someone with whom students have had regular, ongoing contact.

Questions might address how students felt when they learned the person was ill, how they felt at different points in the experience (e.g., when the person went into the hospital for the first/last time, when the person could not come to school any longer), what they are thinking or feeling about these events now.

Close the discussion by acknowledging the feelings students have expressed, validating feelings of sadness, inviting further discussion as a class in the future, and offering one-on-one discussions if they wish (with you or some other school resource, such as a school nurse or counselor).

Family Activity

Distribute Family Activity Sheet 2.3, **Different Ways to Be Sick**, and ask students to complete the sheet with their parents.

How AIDS Works: Grades K–3

Elizabeth and Mrs. Shaw

Elizabeth's head ached. Her throat had really hurt a couple of days ago, so her mother took her to the doctor. The doctor said she had strep throat and would have to stay home from school. The doctor gave her some medicine to help her get better.

This morning, Elizabeth's mother set up a special place in the big chair by the front window and wrapped her in the thick blue quilt her grandma had made. She gave her some fat, soft pillows to lean on. Her picture books were on the table next to her. Her dinosaur puppets were at her feet, and her cat, Max, was sleeping in the corner. She finished drinking the last of her hot chocolate.

Elizabeth felt bored. She was tired of being sick. Her books didn't interest her and her toys were not much fun. She liked sitting by the window, though, because she could see all kinds of things going on outside.

A fat robin landed in the red berry bush and started eating the berries. She saw her friends on their way to school. Mary Helen was riding her new bicycle, and Skip splashed in a puddle and got mud all over himself. She counted 6 red cars and 3 green ones driving down the street. Mr. and Mrs. Shaw, the next door neighbors, walked by.

Mrs. Shaw was very thin and looked tired. She walked slowly, with her hand on Mr. Shaw's arm. The two of them talked and smiled, but every now and then Mrs. Shaw made a face, like something hurt.

Elizabeth's mother came in with her medicine. "Mom," said Elizabeth, "Mrs. Shaw looks like she's sick, too. What's wrong with her?"

"Remember, we talked about Mrs. Shaw having cancer? The medicines they give her for her cancer make her feel very sick. But we hope they'll help her get better, and that she'll be well again. And speaking of medicine, I've got a spoonful here for your sore throat."

Elizabeth swallowed the medicine and crinkled up her nose, even though it didn't really taste that bad.

"When will Mrs. Shaw be better?" she asked her mother.

(continued)

How AIDS Works: Grades K–3

TEACHER PAGE 2.1

continued

"Well, we don't know for sure," her mother answered. "She has a very serious kind of cancer, and she could be sick for a few months. Her medicines may not work as quickly as the doctors would like. She's been home from work for a couple of months now, and I think this could go on for a few more months."

Elizabeth waved to the Shaws as they walked by her window, and they smiled and waved back. She pulled the blue quilt closely around herself and wondered how long *she* would be sick.

A little while later, Elizabeth was surprised to hear someone knocking at the door. Her mother answered, and Mr. Shaw came in with some flowers from his garden. "I noticed you were home sick," he said. "I thought these flowers might cheer you up."

"Thank you," said Elizabeth. "I know Mrs. Shaw is sick, too. My mom says she has been very sick for a long time, and can't go to work."

"That's true, Elizabeth. She's been sick for a while now."

"I'm too sick to go to school. The doctor told me so. But we are learning about rain forests at school now, and I don't want to be sick for a long time. I want to go back to school."

"How long did the doctor say you should stay home?" asked Mr. Shaw.

"I don't know. But I think two months would be way too long for me. I hope I get better sooner than Mrs. Shaw does."

Mr. Shaw smiled. "Oh, I'm sure you will, Elizabeth. Your mom says you have strep throat. That is a very different kind of illness from cancer. If you take your medicine and rest, I think you'll be back at school next week."

"Well, that's good," said Elizabeth. "Why is cancer so different from strep throat?"

"It is a more serious disease," said Mr. Shaw. "It makes the body much sicker than strep throat does. And your medicine works very well and helps your strep throat heal up quickly. The medicines for the cancer Mrs. Shaw has don't always work right away."

"Oh, I have an idea!" said Elizabeth, suddenly excited. "I can share my medicine with Mrs. Shaw. If it works so well for me, it might help her get better, too."

(continued)

TEACHER PAGE 2.1
continued

"What a nice idea, Elizabeth," said Mr. Shaw. "But the medicine the doctor gave you for strep throat is a special medicine just for that illness. It won't help someone with cancer."

Elizabeth looked confused. Mr. Shaw explained some more. "Different illnesses are different for a lot of reasons. There are different ways people get them. And each illness makes people sick in different ways. Strep throat gives you a sore throat, a headache and a fever. The cancer Mrs. Shaw has makes it hard for her to eat and she feels very weak.

"There are also different things people can do to get better from different illnesses," Mr. Shaw continued. "For strep throat, you take the medicine the doctor gave you, and you get lots of rest. You will feel better in a week. But cancer is more serious. Mrs. Shaw takes a different kind of medicine, and it will take her many months to get better."

Elizabeth liked Mr. Shaw, and she felt better after she talked to him. At first, she had been afraid that her strep throat was like Mrs. Shaw's cancer and that she would have to stay home for a long time. Now she understood that the illness she had was different from the one Mrs. Shaw had. But she felt bad for Mrs. Shaw.

"I don't like being sick at all, not even for a week," she told Mr. Shaw. "I'll bet Mrs. Shaw doesn't like being sick for such a long time."

"You're right, Elizabeth, she doesn't. It's hard to feel sick for so long."

"Well, thank you very much for the flowers," said Elizabeth. "Maybe next week, after I get well, I can come down and visit you and Mrs. Shaw."

"We would both like that very much. Thank you," said Mr. Shaw.

After Mr. Shaw left, Elizabeth's mother came in and tucked the blue quilt around her again. Elizabeth felt drowsy and let her eyes drop closed. She must have fallen asleep. In her sleep, she dreamed of rain forests filled with robins, and she saw wild animals splashing around mud puddles and gathering bouquets of beautiful flowers. She had the biggest bouquet of all, and she took it to her friends Mr. and Mrs. Shaw. They could see how strong and healthy she was, carrying that big bunch of flowers, and they smiled and laughed to see her.

© ETR Associates

How AIDS Works: Grades K–3

STUDENT ACTIVITY SHEET 2.2

Name _____

Elizabeth and Mrs. Shaw

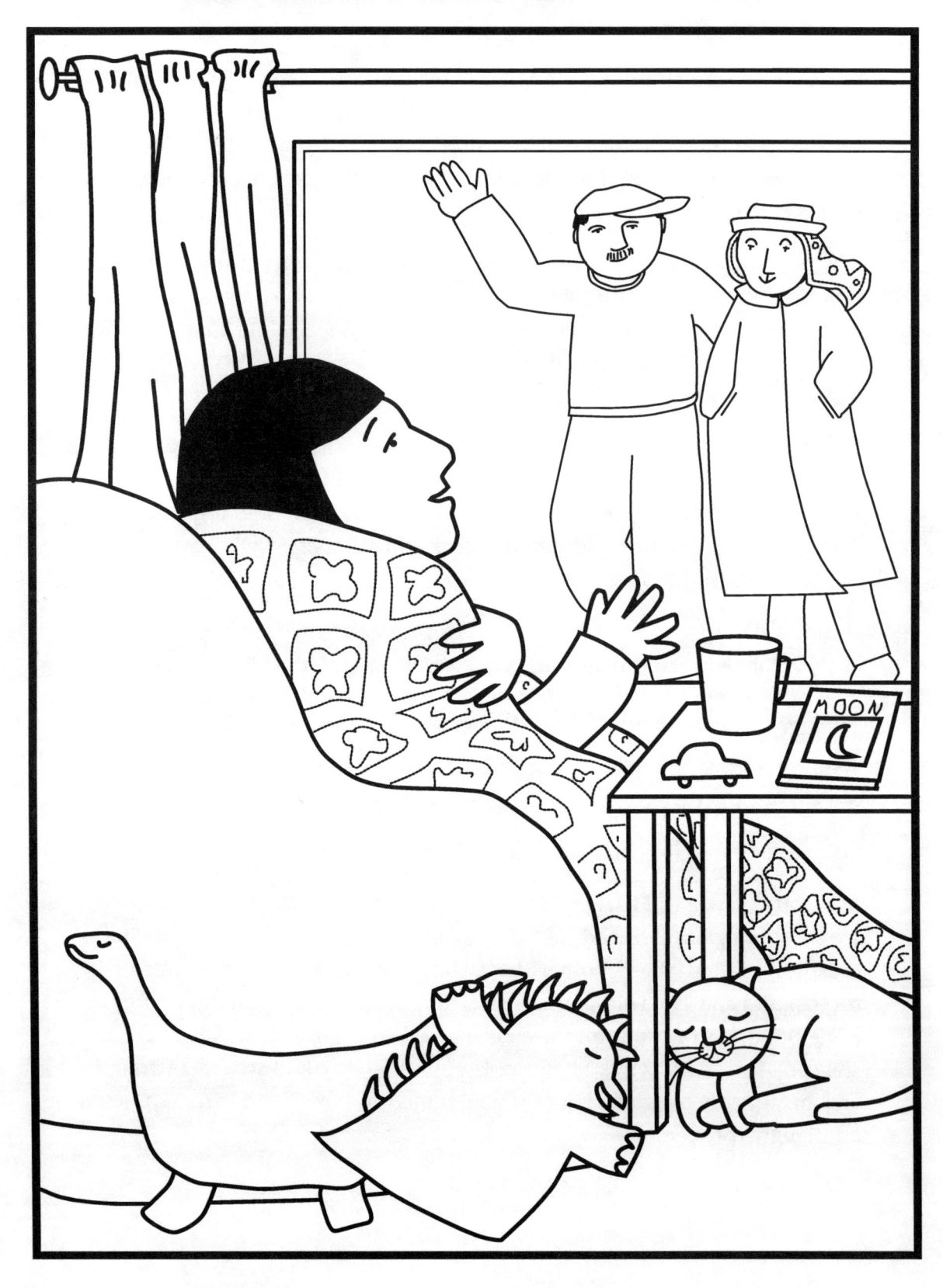

56

Unit 2: Different Ways to Be Sick

FAMILY ACTIVITY SHEET 2.3

Different Ways to Be Sick

Dear Parents,

In Unit 2 of the AIDS curriculum, students are learning to describe some of the differences between type of illnesses. The lessons help them understand that most illnesses children get are not serious.

These are the concepts for Unit 2:

1. Some germs can live in many different places—the air, the surface of a desk, hands, in the body. Other germs can only live in a few places—inside the body, for example.
2. Some communicable illnesses are easy to pass between people. Some are hard to pass.
3. Some illnesses are very serious, and others are not so serious. Some illnesses are hard to treat and others are easy to treat. Most illnesses get better on their own.
4. Most of the illnesses children get are not serious and are easy to treat.

Student Work

As part of these lessons, students listened to a story, "Elizabeth and Mrs. Shaw," about a child with strep throat (a not-so-serious illness) and her neighbor with cancer (a serious illness). They then completed an activity sheet or a drawing.

Please ask your child to show you the activity sheet or drawing. Ask your child the following questions about the lesson (sample answers are provided):

1. What happened in the story about Elizabeth and Mrs. Shaw? What does your activity sheet or drawing show?
2. Elizabeth's illness was not a serious illness. How do we know this?

   She had not been sick for a long time. There were medicines she could take that would help her get better. Her mother and her doctor knew she would get better in a few days. She could help herself get better just by resting and staying at home for a few days.

(continued)

How AIDS Works: Grades K–3

FAMILY ACTIVITY SHEET 2.3
continued

3. Mrs. Shaw's illness was a serious illness. How do we know this?

   She had been very sick and felt very bad. She was sick for a long time. She had been too sick to go to work for a long time. The medicines she was taking did not help her get better right away. Her doctor did not know when she would get better.

4. Let's talk about some of the illnesses we have seen in our family. Have they been serious or not so serious?

   The answer to this question will vary from family to family. Most of the illnesses children get are not serious and are easy to treat. Use this discussion to emphasize this point with your child. However, if your family has been affected by serious illnesses in adults or children, you can also use this opportunity to discuss the experience. You might explore your child's feelings about this and answer any questions.

Further Information

The first 3 units of the curriculum teach about illnesses in general. Beginning in Unit 4, students will be learning specifically about AIDS.

You will not need to have all the facts about AIDS to talk about the topic with your child and respond to questions. If you would like further information about the lessons, please feel free to call me at _____.

If you have questions about AIDS, you can call the National AIDS Hotline at 1-800-342-AIDS, or the local AIDS Hotline at _____.
If your child asks you something about AIDS and you do not know the answer, you could call the hotline together for more information.

Sincerely,

_____
(Teacher name)

Unit 3

How the Body Stays Well

Time 60 minutes

Unit Objective Students will be able to explain how the body protects us from germs, both outside and inside the body.

Concepts
1. A germ cannot make a person sick unless it has some way to get into the body.
2. The body has many ways of protecting itself from germs and healing itself from illness or injury.

Overview Unit 3 builds greater understanding about communicable diseases and the human immune system. It also provides reassurance that the body has many ways to protect itself from germs. Students who master these concepts will understand more clearly, in Units 4 and 5, that AIDS is a serious illness because it affects the body's ability to fight off other illnesses, and that it is a hard-to-pass illness because it is hard for the AIDS germ to get inside the body.

Unit Summary **Activity 1. How Can Germs Get Inside the Body? (10 minutes):** The teacher briefly *reviews* the concepts from earlier units. Then, in an *interactive exercise*, students look at one another and identify 3 portals of entry for germs (eyes, nose, mouth). The teacher explains how the body protects each of these openings from germs.

(continued)

Activity 2. The Body Protects Itself (10 minutes): In a *demonstration,* the teacher shows how the skin of an apple protects it from dirt, but how, when the skin is cut, dirt and germs are able to get inside. The parallel between the apple's skin and human skin is explained.

Activity 3. Inside the Body: Defending the Castle (10 minutes): The teacher tells a *story,* drawing simple pictures on the board, to explain that special helper cells in the blood fight germs that get inside the body.

Activity 4. How Helper Cells Fight Germs (15 minutes): A *demonstration* shows how helper cells in the blood fight germs inside the body. Dramatic effects are achieved using colored water, vinegar and baking soda.

Evaluation. The Immune System at Work (10–15 minutes): Older students *draw* a picture showing the immune system fighting germs to demonstrate their understanding of how the body protects itself. Younger students complete an *activity sheet.*

Family Activity. The *family activity* offers students a chance to discuss the lesson with parents.

Developmental Framework

- Younger students may have more trouble understanding internal body systems, such as the immune system, that help protect the body from disease. Keep explanations simple and concrete. Don't worry if students do not fully comprehend the details. The overall concepts for this unit are well within the cognitive capabilities of younger students, and these are most important.

- An activity sheet is available as an alternative to the drawing activity in the Evaluation.

Terms to Use

- immune system
- helper cells

Review Teacher Content Summaries for Unit 3:
- **Portals of Entry for Germs** (p. 145)
- **Understanding the Immune System** (p. 147)

Get Ready

For Activity 2 have:

- an apple
- pie plate or other flat container filled with soil
- paper towels
- small, sharp knife

For Activity 4 have:

- a clear container with a lid
- water
- stick for stirring
- red food coloring
- baking soda, in a container labeled "helper cells"
- white vinegar, in a clear container labeled "germs"

For Evaluation have:

- drawing materials *(for older students)*
- **How Can Germs Get In?** (Student Activity Sheet 3.1) *(for younger students)*
- **How the Body Stays Well** (Family Activity Sheet 3.2) *(for all students)*

Activity 1

How Can Germs Get Inside the Body?

Time	10 minutes
Objective	Students will be able to identify or describe 3 openings through which germs can enter the body, and a way each of these openings is protected from germs.
Teacher Background	• Portals of Entry for Germs (p. 145)

Review concepts Use the Review Guide (p. 157) to review concepts from earlier units. Areas where students have demonstrated successful understanding of the concepts can be reviewed briefly; review those where concepts may still present a challenge in more depth.

Ask one or more of the questions provided for each previous unit, confirming answers that demonstrate understanding of the concepts and clarifying any misconceptions.

Students look for ways germs can enter the body Explain that for a germ to make a person sick, the germ must have some way to get inside the body.

Have students pair up. Ask students to look at their partners' faces and identify places germs might be able to get inside the body.

Student answers should include eyes, nose and mouth. Students may also mention breaks in the skin or sores.

Describe ears Explain how ears are different from other places germs get inside the body:

- There is a thin piece of skin—the ear drum—at the end of the ear canal (the narrow tunnel in the ear).
- As long as the ear drum is healthy, germs cannot get inside the body through the ears.
- Ear infections are the result of germs that have gotten inside the body through other openings, such as the mouth or nose.

Activity 1   How Can Germs Get Inside the Body? *continued*

Describe how openings are protected

Describe the ways each opening in the body is protected from germs. It is important for students to feel reassured that the body has many ways to protect itself from disease-causing germs.

- **Eyes:** Eyelids and eyebrows protect from dirt and dust. Tears help clean eyes and wash away dirt, dust and germs.
- **Nose:** Hairs in nose keep out dirt, dust and germs. Mucus helps clean out dirt or dust that gets into the nose.
- **Mouth:** Saliva can kill some germs, and can help wash out dirt or dust.
- **Coughing and sneezing:** These actions can help clear dirt, dust and pollen out of the body.
- **Ears:** Tiny hairs and ear wax help keep ear canals free of dirt and dust. The ear drum protects the inside of the body.

Ongoing Assessment

Use the following questions to assess whether students understand that germs must get inside the body to cause illness, can describe the openings through which germs can enter the body, and can explain the natural protections these openings have from germs.

- If a germ cannot get inside the body, can it still make a person sick?

  No, a germ has to get inside the body before it can make a person sick.

- What are some of the ways germs can get inside the body?

  Germs can get into the body through the eyes, nose and mouth.

- What are some of the ways the body keeps germs from getting inside?

  The ear has a thin piece of skin that protects the inside of the body from germs; tiny hairs and ear wax protect the ear canal. Eyes have eyelids and eyebrows, tears. Noses have hairs and mucus. Mouths have saliva that can kill some germs and wash out dust and dirt. Coughing and sneezing can clear out dust, dirt, pollen and germs.

How AIDS Works: Grades K–3

Activity 2

The Body Protects Itself

Time	10 minutes
Objective	Students will be able to understand how skin protects the body from germs and describe how germs can get inside the body through cuts in the skin.
Materials	• apple • pie plate with soil • paper towels • knife

Explain role of skin

Explain to students that one of the most wonderful ways the body has to protect itself from germs is the skin. The entire body is covered with skin, and skin helps keep germs outside the body.

Demonstrate how skin protects the body

Hold up the apple. Tell the following story to students, performing the actions as indicated:

Imagine this apple is a child playing outside.

Rub the apple in the plate of soil.

Look! The child is getting covered in dirt as she plays.

Hold up the apple and show how the soil adheres to the skin.

Now she has dirt all over. What should she do?

Encourage answers that suggest the child wash off with soap and water. Wipe the apple clean with a paper towel.

Yes, she can clean the dirt off with soap and water. I'll use a paper towel now, but soap and water would work even better.

Explain how the skin protects the apple:

The apple has a skin, just like a person does. The apple's skin keeps dirt—and germs—outside the apple's body the same way human skin keeps dirt and germs outside a child's body.

Activity 2   The Body Protects Itself, *continued*

Demonstrate how germs can get inside the body

Make a small vertical cut in the apple and remove a wedge.

Let's suppose there's a cut in the skin. What if the child goes out to play now?

Rub the apple in the soil again and then show it to the class. Wipe it clean with a paper towel. Soil will remain in the cut section.

You can see that dirt and germs are able to get inside the body now.

Cut a larger horizontal wedge from the apple to show how the dirt is inside the apple only in the area underneath the original cut. Pass the apple around so the class can see it, or have one student carry the apple around the room.

Explain that this is why people with a cut should wash the wound with soap and water, and cover it with a bandage. Then dirt and germs cannot get inside the body.

Discuss how the body heals itself

Ask if anyone has ever had a cut or a scrape. What was this like? How long did it take to heal? Emphasize that the body has wonderful ways to heal itself from illness and injuries, and that most students have seen this at work many times in their own bodies.

Ongoing Assessment

Use the following questions to assess whether students understand how germs can get inside the body through cuts in the skin, and that intact skin protects the body from germs.

- If you get a cut in your skin, what can happen?

    Germs can get inside the body through the cut.

- If there are no cuts or openings in the skin, what happens to germs on the skin?

    If there are no cuts in the skin, germs can be washed off. Germs can't get inside through the skin. Germs could get inside through the mouth or nose, but not through the skin.

How AIDS Works: Grades K–3

Activity 3

Inside the Body: Defending the Castle

Time	10 minutes
Objective	Students will be able to explain that special helper cells in the blood help the body fight germs.
Teacher Background	• Understanding the Immune System (p. 147)

■ **Note:** Younger students, especially in kindergarten and first grade, have a limited ability to understand internal body processes generally, and the subtleties of the human immune system are well beyond their understanding. However, they are fascinated by the ways the body works and will enjoy information about how the body protects itself from disease.

In this activity, a simplified presentation of the immune system is offered. Students will be able to grasp the idea that there are elements in blood called "helper cells" that fight disease. This is really the essential concept for the activity, and more sophisticated knowledge is not necessary.

Introduce immune system

Remind students that they have talked about many of the ways the body protects itself from germs. These have included some "outside" ways—things on the outside of the body like skin or hair—that keep germs from getting inside the body.

Explain that when germs *do* get inside the body, the body has some "inside" ways to protect itself.

These "inside ways" the body protects itself are part of something called the "immune system." The body's immune system helps people stay healthy by fighting germs that get inside the body.

Activity 3   Inside the Body: Defending the Castle, *continued*

Describe blood   Explain that one of the important tools the body uses to keep itself strong and protect itself from germs that get inside the body is blood. Ask students to volunteer information about blood ("What do you know about blood?"). The goal is simply to get a range of answers that describe aspects of blood. Validate students' responses.

> **Note:** Younger students may have more trouble volunteering information. You may need to fill in some answers for them.

Possible answers:

- Blood is red.
- Blood is pumped by the heart.
- You can see blood if you cut yourself.
- Blood carries oxygen throughout the body.
- Everyone has blood.
- People need blood to live.

Explain that blood is made up of a lot of different things which cannot be seen without a microscope. Cells are the smallest part of the blood. The blood includes special cells called "helper cells." These helper cells fight germs and help keep the body healthy.

Tell a story to explain how the immune system works   Tell students the following story, illustrating on the board as indicated.

Imagine that you are in charge of a big castle.

Draw a simple castle on the board.

You have built a big wall around the castle.

Draw a big circle around the castle to represent the wall.

> *This wall is so high and so strong, most invaders are unable to attack the castle. Once in a while, however, a group of invaders does manage to get over the wall. Imagine a group of them now, getting ready to attack your castle.*

Draw some stick figures of invaders inside the wall of the castle.

> *Luckily for you, you have a group of special defenders of the castle.*

(continued)

How AIDS Works: Grades K–3

Activity 3   **Inside the Body: Defending the Castle,** *continued*

> *As soon as they see the invaders, they run out, confront them, overcome them and kill them.*

Draw some stick figures of "special defenders" confronting the invaders. Erase the invaders.

> *Now the castle is safe!*

Explain helper cells   Explain that this story also describes the way helper cells in the blood help defend the body from germs. Using the pictures on the board, tell the following story:

> *Imagine that this castle is really your body. The big wall around the castle is your skin. Now some invaders—germs—get past your skin and inside your body. Remember how this might happen— through your mouth, nose, eyes, or cuts in your skin.*

Draw some stick figures of invaders again, inside the wall.

> *Lucky for you, your blood has special cells called "helper cells" that know how to fight this kind of invader. As soon as they see the invader germs, the helper cells confront the germs and kill them.*

Point to the defenders—the "helper cells"—in the drawing, and erase the invaders.

> *Even though these germs got inside the body, the body was able to fight them off. Most of the time when germs are able to get inside our bodies, helper cells in our blood kill the germs before they can make us sick.*
>
> *Once in a while, helper cells are not able to fight off all the germs. Then they have to call in more helper cells. When this happens, your body might get sick. After a few days, the body's defenders— the immune system—are usually able to fight off all the germs, and you start to feel better again.*
>
> *Helper cells are also called "white blood cells."*

Activity 3   Inside the Body: Defending the Castle, *continued*

Check students' understanding Ask questions to check students' understanding. Explain that in the next activity, the class will learn more about how helper cells in the blood fight germs.

Ongoing Assessment Use the following question to assess whether students understand that blood helps play a role in fighting germs and keeping the body healthy.

- How does blood help the body fight germs?

   Special helper cells in the blood fight germs.

Activity 4

How Helper Cells Fight Germs

Time	15 minutes
Objective	Students will be able to explain how helper cells fight germs and that things that happen inside the body and can't be seen are very important in keeping people healthy.
Materials	• clear container with a lid • water • stick for stirring • red food coloring • baking soda, in a container labeled "helper cells" • white vinegar, in a clear container labeled "germs"

Perform demonstration Tell students you are going to give them an idea of how helper cells protect the body from germs.

Fill the clear container with about 1 inch of tap water. Put the lid in place. Show this container to students. Point to the outside of the container as you begin the demonstration.

> *Let's pretend that this container is a body. This body has a skin. Germs cannot get inside the body unless there is a cut in the body, or unless they enter through an opening such as the mouth.*

Take off the lid of the container.

> *Remember, we talked about how important cells in the blood are in helping to fight germs that get inside the body?*

Add a small amount of food coloring to the container, until the water is dark red.

> *We're adding some color to show the blood inside this body. This is really just food coloring, but it gives us the idea that there is blood here.*

Add a heaping teaspoon of baking soda from the container marked "helper cells." Mix the soda in until it is dissolved and not visible.

(continued)

Activity 4 How Helper Cells Fight Germs, *continued*

Now we're adding some pretend helper cells to this blood. Once they're mixed in, we cannot see these helper cells. Sometimes, these helper cells are called "white blood cells."

You cannot see the helper cells without a microscope. Even though we cannot see the helper cells, they are there, waiting to protect the body.

Close the lid of the container and hold it up for students to see.

Now we have our pretend body with skin protecting it on the outside and blood protecting it on the inside. But imagine that somehow some germs get inside this body. Remember how this could happen?—through the mouth, nose, eyes or cuts in the skin.

Pick up the bottle of vinegar labeled "germs."

In this bottle, we have some pretend germs. Can you see them? Germs are so small you can't see them. What do you think will happen if some of these germs get into this body?

Open the container. Pour a small amount of the vinegar into the container and mix gently. The mixture will fizz.

The helper cells in the blood are fighting off the germs!

Explain that while this demonstration did not use real germs or blood, it gives students an idea of how helper cells in the blood can fight germs.

Discuss internal body process Discuss with students the idea of internal processes (things that happen inside the body) that cannot be seen, but are still very important in keeping us healthy. Ask if students can think of other important things that happen in the body that cannot be seen.

Possible answers:
- digesting food
- eliminating wastes
- growing (getting taller, hair and nails growing)
- getting tired, sleeping, and waking up with energy for a new day

How AIDS Works: Grades K–3

Activity 4   **How Helper Cells Fight Germs,** *continued*

Ongoing Assessment

Use the following questions to assess whether students understand that helper cells in the blood keep the body healthy, and that these helper cells are one of many internal processes that cannot be seen but are very important in keeping people healthy.

- What do the helper cells do when they find germs in the blood? In our demonstration they "fizzed." What were the cells doing when they fizzed?

    Helper cells fight germs that get into the body; they attack germs and kill them.

- What are some things that happen inside the body, that we cannot see, that help keep us healthy?

    Helper cells fight germs; hair, nails and bodies grow; food is digested; wastes are eliminated; people get tired, rest and wake up with new energy.

Evaluation

The Immune System at Work

Time	10–15 minutes
Objective	Students will be able to demonstrate that they understand that germs must get into the body to make a person sick and how the immune system works to fight germs that get inside the body.
Materials	• How Can Germs Get In? (3.1) OR drawing materials • How the Body Stays Well (3.2)

Students complete assignment

For younger students:

Distribute Student Activity Sheet 3.1, **How Can Germs Get In?**.

Ask students to circle pictures that show ways germs can get into the body. Ask them to draw an "X" through pictures that do not show ways germs can get into the body.

When students have finished, review and discuss the activity sheet to check comprehension.

For older students:

Distribute drawing materials. Ask students to draw a picture showing the immune system fighting germs. This might be a picture of special helper cells in the blood fighting germs. It could also be a fantasy picture of a strong being, representing helper cells or the immune system, fighting disease-causing germs.

Students with writing skills could also write a short essay describing what their picture shows.

Discuss students' drawings to check comprehension.

Family Activity

Distribute Family Activity Sheet 3.2, **How the Body Stays Well**. Ask students to take their drawings or activity sheets home and discuss their work with their parents.

How AIDS Works: Grades K–3

STUDENT ACTIVITY SHEET 3.1

Name _____

How Can Germs Get In?

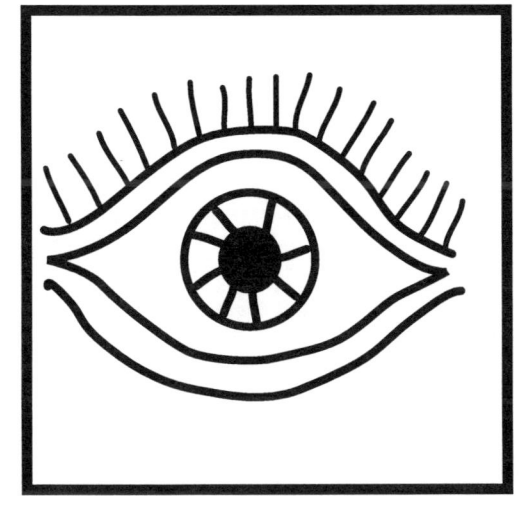

eye

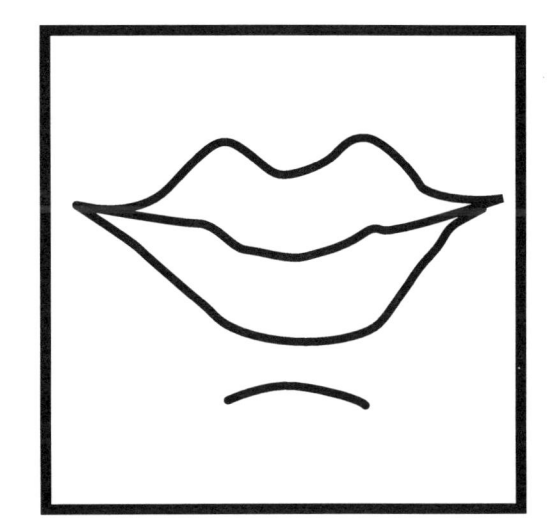

mouth

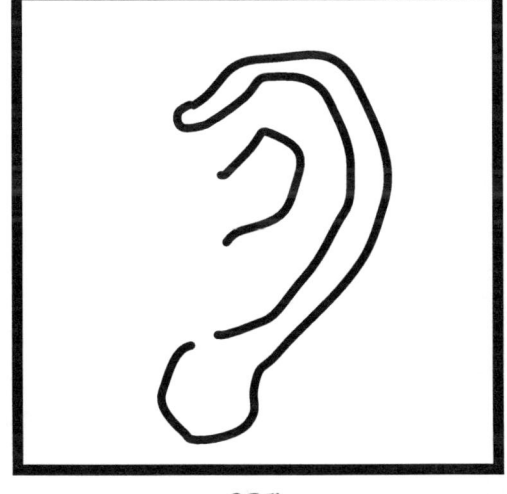

ear

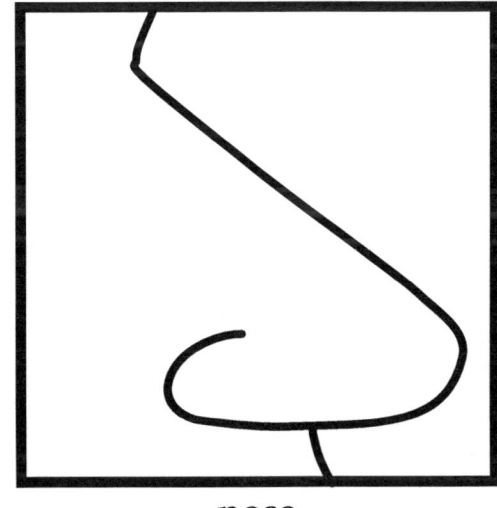

nose

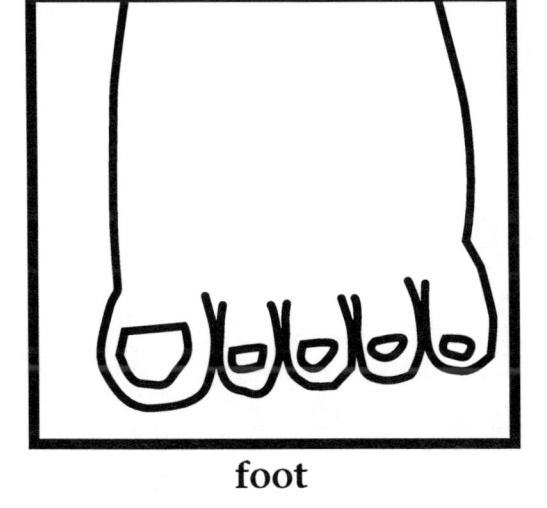

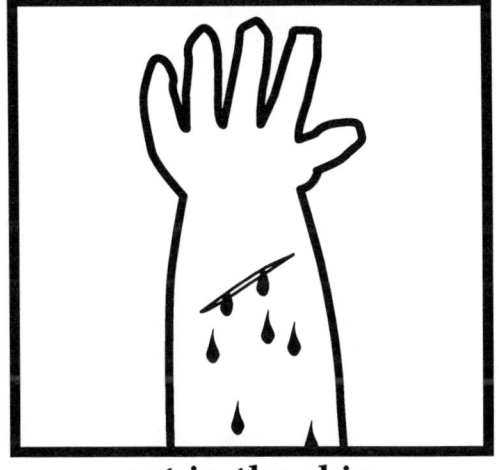

foot

cut in the skin

© ETR Associates

How AIDS Works: Grades K–3

75

FAMILY ACTIVITY SHEET 3.2

How the Body Stays Well

Dear Parents,

In Unit 3 of the AIDS curriculum, students are learning how the body protects us from germs, both outside and inside the body.

These are the concepts for Unit 3:

1. A germ cannot make a person sick unless it gets into the body.
2. The body has many ways of protecting itself from germs and healing itself from illness.

Student Work

As part of these lessons, students either completed an activity sheet or a drawing. If your child has an activity sheet, ask what it shows. You can also ask questions 1 and 2. If your child has a drawing, ask about the drawing and what it shows. You can also ask questions 3 and 4.

Activity Sheet:

1. There are 3 important body openings—eyes, nose and mouth. Are there ways these body openings can keep germs out?

   Your child should be able to identify one way each of these body openings keeps germs out. Possible answers:

   - *Eyes: Eyelids and eyebrows protect from dirt and dust. Tears help clean eyes and wash away dirt, dust and germs.*
   - *Nose: Hairs in nose keep out dirt, dust and germs. Mucus helps clean out dirt or dust that gets into the nose.*
   - *Mouth: Saliva can kill some germs, and can help wash out dirt or dust.*
   - *Coughing and sneezing can help clear dirt, dust and pollen out of the body.*

© ETR Associates

How AIDS Works: Grades K–3

FAMILY ACTIVITY SHEET 3.2

continued

2. What makes ears different from the eyes, nose and mouth?

   A thin piece of skin, the ear drum, is at the end of the opening of the ear. This keeps dirt, dust and germs from getting inside the head through the ears. Tiny hairs and ear wax help keep ear canals free of dirt and dust. This keeps the ear drum healthy.

Drawing:

3. What is the most interesting thing you learned about how the body fights germs?

4. Can you think of a time your own immune system helped protect your body from germs?

Further Information

The first 3 units of the curriculum teach about illnesses in general. Beginning in Unit 4, students will be learning specifically about AIDS.

You will not need to have all the facts about AIDS to talk about the topic with your child and respond to questions. If you would like further information about the lessons, please feel free to call me at _____.

If you have questions about AIDS, you can call the National AIDS Hotline at 1-800-342-AIDS, or the local AIDS Hotline at _____.
If your child asks you something about AIDS and you do not know the answer, you could call the hotline together for more information.

Sincerely,

_____
(Teacher name)

Unit 4

What About AIDS?

Time 70 minutes

Unit Objective Students will be able to explain why AIDS is hard to pass from one person to another and understand that children don't have to worry about getting it.

Concepts
1. The AIDS germ is an "inside germ." It is not easily passed from one person to another.

2. The AIDS germ can only be passed from one person to another through a few activities, and most students in elementary school do not do these things. This is why they do not need to worry about having or getting AIDS.

3. The AIDS germ damages the immune system. This makes it hard for the body to fight off diseases.

Overview Unit 4 gives students specific information about HIV and AIDS, with an emphasis on the concepts that HIV is hard to pass from one person to another and does not commonly affect children. The overall focus of this unit is on information. In communities that have been significantly affected by AIDS, however, it may be helpful to talk with students about their feelings concerning AIDS and ways it has affected their lives or the lives of people they know. Optional discussion questions are provided.

(continued)

Unit Summary

Activity 1. About AIDS (15–25 minutes): After a brief *review* of concepts from earlier units, the teacher asks students what they know or have heard about AIDS and leads a *discussion* to provide general information. The concept of "inside" germs (germs that live in the blood and certain other fluids inside the body) is introduced. Optional *discussion questions* explore students' feelings about AIDS.

Activity 2. Keeping "Inside" Germs Outside (10 minutes): Using containers with colored water and clear water, the teacher *demonstrates* that skin keeps "inside" germs from passing from one person to another.

Activity 3. How Is AIDS Passed? (10 minutes): In a brief *lecture,* the teacher explains that AIDS can only be passed in a few ways.

Activity 4: What Does the AIDS Germ Do to the Body? (10 minutes): The earlier *demonstration* (from Unit 3) that used baking soda and vinegar to show helper cells "fizzing" when germs got into the blood is revisited. This time it is used to show helper cells not working.

Evaluation. AIDS Is Hard to Get (10–15 minutes): To demonstrate their understanding of how the AIDS germ works, older students *draw* a picture showing some of the activities people can do together that present no risk of HIV transmission. Younger students complete an *activity sheet* identifying things people can do together that present no risk of HIV transmission.

Family Activity. The *family activity* offers students a chance to discuss the lesson with their parents.

Developmental Framework

- Younger students may have less information to volunteer in Activity 1. You may need to fill in this discussion.

- For younger students in Activity 4, revisit the concept presented in Unit 3 about internal processes that cannot be seen, but are still very important in keeping us healthy.

- An activity sheet is available as an alternative to the drawing activity in the Evaluation.

- Older students may be able to distinguish between AIDS and HIV: HIV is the name of the germ (virus) that causes AIDS. Anyone infected with HIV has HIV infection and many people with HIV look and feel healthy. AIDS is usually only diagnosed at an advanced stage of HIV infection, and most people with AIDS

(continued)

have had some serious health problems. This distinction is not essential to the lesson, however.

- Older students may also be comfortable with the more precise term "AIDS virus" rather than the more generic "AIDS germ."

Terms to Use
- AIDS
- "inside" germ
- fluids inside the body
- transfusion
- injection drug use

Review Teacher Content Summaries for Unit 4:
- **3 Points About AIDS** (p. 149)
- **Talking About AIDS Transmission with Early Elementary Students** (p. 150)
- **Children's Understanding of Drugs and AIDS** (p. 151)

Get Ready *For Activity 2 have:*
- 2 clear containers with lids
- water
- blue food coloring

For Activity 4 have:
- a clear container with a lid
- water
- stick for stirring
- red food coloring
- white vinegar, in a clear container labeled "germs"

For Evaluation have:
- **AIDS Is Hard to Get** (Student Activity Sheet 4.1) *(for younger students)*
- drawing materials *(for older students)*
- **What About AIDS?** (Family Activity Sheet 4.2) *(for all students)*

How AIDS Works: Grades K–3

Activity 1

About AIDS

Time	15 minutes (plus additional 5–10 minutes for optional discussion)
Objective	Students will be able to explain that the AIDS germ is different from other germs because it is an "inside" germ.
Teacher Background	• 3 Points About AIDS (p. 149)

■ **Note:** In communities that have been significantly affected by AIDS, children may have many emotional concerns. If students have relatives or friends affected, or if there are students or teachers in the school known to have HIV or AIDS, you may want to spend some time talking about thoughts and feelings. Optional discussion questions are provided.

Review concepts

Use the Review Guide (p. 157) to review concepts from earlier units. Areas where students have demonstrated successful understanding of the concepts can be reviewed briefly; review those where concepts may still present a challenge in more depth.

Ask one or more of the questions provided for each previous unit, confirming answers that demonstrate understanding of the concepts and clarifying any misconceptions.

Students brainstorm what they know about AIDS

Explain that the class will be talking about AIDS in this lesson, and that they will begin by discussing some of the things they already know or have heard about the disease.

Ask students:

What are some of the things you know or have heard about AIDS? These can be facts you are sure of, or things you have heard and are not sure about.

(continued)

Activity 1 About AIDS, *continued*

Gather a range of responses. Acknowledge student contributions without correcting or expanding. For older students who can read, list comments on the board.

Provide correct information about AIDS

Using student responses as a starting point, provide further information about AIDS and correct any misunderstandings. Try, in particular, to cover the following issues:

- AIDS is important because it is a serious disease that is affecting many people's lives.

- The AIDS germ is different from other kinds of germs. It is an "inside" germ—it only lives in the blood and other special fluids inside the body.

- The AIDS germ does not pass from person to person in the easy way colds or flus do. AIDS is hard to get.

- While some children do have AIDS, it is not a common disease among children.

Try to touch on all of the student responses. Some might be addressed directly by this activity. Others may be discussed in more detail later in the unit.

(Optional) Discuss feelings about AIDS

Invite students to discuss their feelings about AIDS and how it has affected their lives. Possible questions to guide this discussion:

- Do you ever have thoughts about AIDS? What kinds of things do you think about?

- How do you feel when you hear about someone who has AIDS?

- Does AIDS ever make you worry about things? What kinds of things?

Offer validation and understanding for students' feelings, and reassurance where possible for their concerns. Remember that many children have unreasonable fears that they have AIDS or are at risk for AIDS. Simple statements of reassurance in response to children's comments can help lighten such anxieties.

(continued)

Activity 1 **About AIDS,** *continued*

Example:

> *It is natural for people to worry about AIDS. It's a scary illness. It is also important for you to know that AIDS is hard to get, and that children your age almost never get infected with the AIDS germ.*

Offer students an opportunity to talk with you after class if they have concerns they wish to speak about privately.

Ongoing Assessment Use the following question to assess whether students understand that AIDS is passed from person to person in different ways from other illnesses and that the AIDS germ is different from other germs.

- What makes the AIDS germ different from other germs?

    The AIDS germ does not pass from person to person in the easy way colds or flus do. The AIDS germ is hard to get.

Activity 2

Keeping "Inside" Germs Outside

Time	10 minutes
Objective	Students will be able to explain that skin helps keep the AIDS germ, an "inside" germ, from getting inside someone else's body.
Materials	• 2 clear containers with lids • water • blue food coloring

Introduce activity Explain that in the last lesson (Unit 3), students learned that for a germ to make a person sick, the germ must have some way to get into the body. In this activity, students are going to learn more about why the AIDS germ is different from other germs, and more about why AIDS is a hard disease to get.

Review how germs are passed Ask students:

What are some ways germs can pass from person to person?

Look for student responses such as coughing, sharing a cup, kissing, getting germs on hands and then touching mouth, and so on.

Explain how AIDS is different Tell students:

Some of the germs we have talked about so far can be passed easily from one person to another. Many of these germs can live in the air, on a cup or fork, or in tiny droplets of saliva or mucus.

The AIDS germ is different. The AIDS germ can only live in blood and other special fluids inside the body. It can only be passed when blood or these other "inside" fluids get out of one person's body and inside another person's body. The AIDS germ cannot live on our skin, it cannot live in the air, and it cannot go through healthy skin.

(continued)

Activity 2 Keeping "Inside" Germs Outside, *continued*

The AIDS germ cannot be passed easily from one person to another. It is not spread by coughing and sneezing, kissing, sharing cups or touching someone. This is why we can be close to someone with AIDS, touch or hug that person, and not catch AIDS the way we might catch a cold.

Demonstrate how skin keeps the AIDS germ inside the body

Take 2 clear containers with lids on, each filled with about 2 inches of water. Color the water in one container dark blue with food coloring. Tell this story about the containers:

Imagine that these containers are 2 friends. One of them, Daryl, has AIDS. We'll pretend that the blue water shows that the AIDS germ is inside Daryl's body.

The other person, Jennifer, does not have AIDS. The water is clear.

Rub the containers together.

Daryl and Jennifer can play together, touch each other and hug each other without spreading the AIDS germ. That's because the AIDS germ is an "inside germ." It cannot pass through skin, the same way the water in these containers cannot pass through the wall of the container.

The AIDS germ is not passed to others by coughing, sneezing, sharing cups, sharing bathrooms or kissing.

People can only catch the AIDS germ from other people who already have the germ inside their body. No one could catch the AIDS germ from Jennifer because she does not have the germ inside her body.

Someone might get the AIDS germ from Daryl, but only if one of the body fluids with the germ gets out of his body and inside another person's body.

Tell students that you will be discussing exactly how the AIDS germ does pass from one person to another in the next activity.

Activity 2   Keeping "Inside" Germs Outside, *continued*

Ongoing Assessment   Use the following questions to assess whether students understand that the AIDS germ is an "inside germ" and that skin protects people from this kind of germ entering the body.

- What makes the AIDS germ different from other germs we have discussed?

    The AIDS germ is an "inside germ." It lives inside the body and cannot live outside the body the way other germs do.

- What is an important way the body is protected from the AIDS germ—something we discussed today?

    The skin keeps inside germs from getting out of one person's body and into another person's body; the AIDS germ cannot pass through healthy skin.

Activity 3

How Is AIDS Passed?

Time	10 minutes
Objective	Students will be able to explain that AIDS is hard to get, that people can only get it in a few ways, and that children do not commonly get AIDS.
Teacher Background	• Talking About AIDS Transmission with Early Elementary Students (p. 150)
	• Children's Understanding of Drugs and AIDS (p. 151)

■ **Note:** This activity may be the most "delicate" of the lesson sequence. It is important to communicate the ideas and facts in this activity in a simple, concrete and direct manner.

Frank discussions of human sexuality can be understood even by very young children when delivered in a clear, age-appropriate manner. When deciding how much detail to offer in this unit, your guiding principles should be your school or district guidelines, your students' expressed interest and your own comfort level.

Review how "outside" germs can spread

Review with students the idea that some kinds of germs can be spread in "outside" ways. For example, a cold can be spread through coughs. The cold germ lives in tiny droplets of saliva that enter the air when someone coughs, and get into other people's bodies through the nose or mouth when they breathe.

Other "outside" ways include sneezes, sharing eating utensils, or touching a surface with germs on it and then touching your mouth.

Activity 3   How Is AIDS Passed? *continued*

Explain how the AIDS germ can spread   Tell students that there are only 4 ways the AIDS germ can be spread from one person to another. Each way is an "inside" way. Describe these ways as follows.

1. Blood-to-Blood Contact

Because the AIDS germ lives in blood, it can be passed between people if blood is passed between them for any reason.

- **Cuts and scrapes:** *If someone who has the AIDS germ is bleeding and that person's blood gets into a cut on someone else's body, then the AIDS germ could be passed.*

    If you are around someone who is bleeding, get a grown-up to help. Try not to touch anyone else's blood. If you do get blood on you for any reason, wash it off with soap and water. Remember, the AIDS germ cannot get through skin that isn't cut or scraped.

    If you have a cut or scrape, you should clean the wound and put a bandage on it. Get a grown-up to help if it is a bad cut or there is a lot of blood.

- **Blood brothers and sisters:** *You may have heard of people who want to show what good friends they are by becoming a "blood brother" or "blood sister." They cut themselves and rub the cuts together. This is not a safe thing to do. There are many better ways to show you care for someone, ways that won't spread the AIDS germ or other germs.*

- **Transfusions:** *Sometimes people need to be given more blood after an accident or during an operation when they have lost a lot of blood. A doctor or nurse may give them some of another person's blood. This is called a "blood transfusion."*

    If the person who gave the blood had the AIDS germ in his or her body, the person who received the blood would probably get AIDS. Because of this, doctors test blood before they give it to anyone else, so the chances of getting AIDS from a blood transfusion are very, very small.

2. Mother-to-Baby Transmission

If a woman who has the AIDS germ gets pregnant, there is a chance her baby will also get the AIDS germ. The baby might get the AIDS germ when it is inside the mother, or while it is being born.

(continued)

Activity 3 **How Is AIDS Passed?** *continued*

Many babies of mothers with the AIDS germ do not get the AIDS germ inside their bodies.

Once a baby is born, he or she is safe from AIDS. Mothers do not pass the AIDS germ to children after they are born. This is why it is OK for a mother or father who has the AIDS germ to keep taking care of her or his children.

3. Close Sexual Contact

If a person has close sexual contact with another person who has the AIDS germ, the first person might also get AIDS.

When I say "close sexual contact," I do not mean things like kissing, hugging or holding hands. We do not need to worry about catching AIDS from these things.

Remember, a cold germ lives in saliva (in the mouth), and a cold can be spread between two people kissing. When one person kisses another, they might share a little saliva.

But kissing does not spread the AIDS germ. The AIDS germ lives in blood and other inside fluids, and people do not share these when they kiss.

4. Sharing Needles for Taking Drugs

Some people use needles to take drugs. If people share needles with someone who has the AIDS germ, they might get the AIDS germ too.

Review content and reassure students. Point out to them that the behaviors that spread the AIDS germ are not the kinds of things children their age usually do. This is why AIDS is not a threat to young children.

Discuss AIDS and needle use Let students know that many people, especially children, are confused about how the AIDS germ can be spread by people who use needles for taking drugs. Tell them you will spend a few moments now explaining how this happens.

Ask students to name some of the different kinds of needles they have heard about or seen. Help expand the list if students do not have many answers.

(continued)

Activity 3   **How Is AIDS Passed?** *continued*

Examples:

- sewing needles (different kinds)
- medical needles (syringes for shots, needles for sewing stitches after an injury)
- tattoo needles
- needles for piercing ears
- needles used for taking drugs

Ask students to remember where the AIDS germ lives. Look for the response "in the blood or in special fluids inside the body." Then ask which of these kinds of needles might get blood on them.

Affirm that any needle that goes through skin can come in contact with blood. That means that it might also come in contact with the AIDS germ, if the person had the AIDS germ inside his or her body. This is why sharing any kind of needle that has come in contact with someone else's blood is dangerous.

Explain that sewing needles are not a usually a problem, unless they have been used for tattooing or piercing ears. Stress that needles used for piercing ears or making tattoos should not be shared.

Reassure students about shots. Needles used by doctors and nurses are clean (sterile). They have never been used before on anyone else, and after they are used once they are thrown away in a special container.

Remind students not to touch or pick up used drug needles they might see. The needles are very sharp and it is easy to get stuck by accident. The AIDS germ or other germs might be on or in the needle. Instead, they should tell a grown-up about the needle.

Clarify that drugs do not cause AIDS

Clarify for students that it is not the drugs that cause AIDS. It is the blood that remains on or inside the drug needle that carries the AIDS germ from the inside of one person's body to the inside of another person's body. Drugs themselves may make a person very sick, but they do not cause AIDS. Drugs that are *not* taken by needles (such as marijuana, cigarettes or alcohol) may make people sick in other ways, but you cannot get AIDS from these drugs.

Activity 3   How Is AIDS Passed? *continued*

Summarize and check comprehension

Explain to students that the lessons in this unit have shown that the AIDS germ is different from other germs, that AIDS does not pass easily from person to person, and that AIDS is hard to get. They have been able to see that children their age do not usually do the kinds of things that might expose them to the AIDS germ. In the next lesson, they will learn more about what the AIDS germ does when it gets into the body and the steps people can take to make sure they do not get AIDS.

Remind students that people can only catch the AIDS germ from someone who already has the AIDS germ in his or her body, and that there are only a few ways this can happen.

Emphasize that very few young children get AIDS. Young children who have the AIDS virus probably got it before they were born. They did not get it from being around another child with AIDS, or a grown-up with AIDS. Students do not need to worry about being around people who have the AIDS germ.

Respond appropriately to any questions students might have.

Ongoing Assessment

Use the following question to assess whether students understand that the AIDS germ is spread in limited ways, and that the disease is hard to get.

- Why do we say the AIDS germ is hard to get?

    There are only a few ways people can get the AIDS germ. The AIDS germ lives inside the body and you can't get it in "outside the body" ways like other germs. Children don't usually do the kinds of things that pass the AIDS germ.

Activity 4

What Does the AIDS Germ Do to the Body?

Time	10 minutes
Objective	Students will reinforce earlier knowledge about how the AIDS germ makes people sick, and be able to describe what happens when helper cells damaged by the AIDS germ do not work.
Materials	• clear container with a lid • water • stick for stirring • red food coloring • white vinegar, in a clear container labeled "germs"

Introduce activity

Remind students of the earlier activity (in Unit 3) that showed how helper cells fought germs that got into the body. Tell them that now you are going to show them one of the reasons the AIDS germ is a special kind of germ, and why AIDS is a very serious disease.

Review how helper cells work

Review with students the work of the helper cells in fighting illness. Ask for a volunteer to describe what the helper cells do.

Confirm responses that describe helper cells identifying and then fighting germs that get inside the body. Students might use the castle analogy, or talk about how the helper cells make the blood "fizz" when germs get inside the body.

Explain to students that when AIDS germs get into the body, they attack the helper cells. Over time, more and more of the helper cells are damaged, and they are no longer able to fight other germs that get inside the body.

How AIDS Works: Grades K–3

Activity 4   What Does the AIDS Germ Do to the Body? *continued*

Demonstrate damaged helper cells

Show students the clear container with about 1 inch of tap water inside it and the lid in place.

> *Once again, we're going to pretend that this container is a body.*

Take off the lid.

> *There are important cells in the blood—helper cells—that help fight germs that get inside the body.*

Add a small amount of red food coloring, until the water is a dark red.

> *Once again, this is just food coloring. But we're going to pretend the red water is blood in this body. We're also going to imagine that the blood in this body has the AIDS germ in it. The AIDS germ has attacked this body's helper cells.*

Pick up the container of vinegar labeled "germs."

> *Here are some pretend germs. There are many different kinds of germs in here. We can't see them because they are too small. What do you think will happen if some of these germs get into this body?*

Students may say the "blood" is going to fizz, or they may understand that, without the helper cells, it will not.

Open the lid of the container. Pour in a small amount of vinegar and mix gently. Nothing will happen.

> *Last time we did this, the blood "fizzed" because the helper cells were fighting off the germs. But this time, the AIDS germ has damaged the helper cells. They can no longer fight off other germs. These other germs now can get into the body and make the person very sick.*

Remind students that the demonstration did not use real germs or blood.

Activity 4   What Does the AIDS Germ Do to the Body? *continued*

Ongoing Assessment Use the following questions to assess whether students understand that the AIDS germ makes people sick by damaging their helper cells so they are unable to fight other germs.

■ What happens to the helper cells if the AIDS germ gets inside a person's body?

They can't "fizz."

■ If the helper cells aren't fizzing, what does that mean?

The cells are damaged and cannot fight germs. When germs invade the body, the helper cells cannot fight them off, and the person gets sick.

How AIDS Works: Grades K–3

Evaluation

AIDS Is Hard to Get

Time	10–15 minutes
Objective	Students will be able to explain that AIDS is hard to pass from one person to another and that children don't have to worry about getting it.
Materials	• AIDS Is Hard to Get (4.1) OR drawing materials • What About AIDS? (4.2)

Students complete assignment

For younger students:

Distribute Student Activity Sheet 4.1, **AIDS Is Hard to Get**.

Ask students to circle pictures that show things people can do together that do not spread AIDS. (All activities pictured are safe.)

When students have finished, discuss responses to check comprehension.

For older students:

Distribute drawing materials. Ask students to draw a picture showing some of the things people can do together that do not spread AIDS. Students with writing skills could also write a short essay describing what their picture shows.

Display students' drawings and discuss to check comprehension.

Family Activity

Distribute Family Activity Sheet 4.2, **What About AIDS?** Ask students to take their drawings or activity sheets home and discuss their work with their parents.

STUDENT ACTIVITY SHEET 4.1

Name _____

AIDS Is Hard to Get

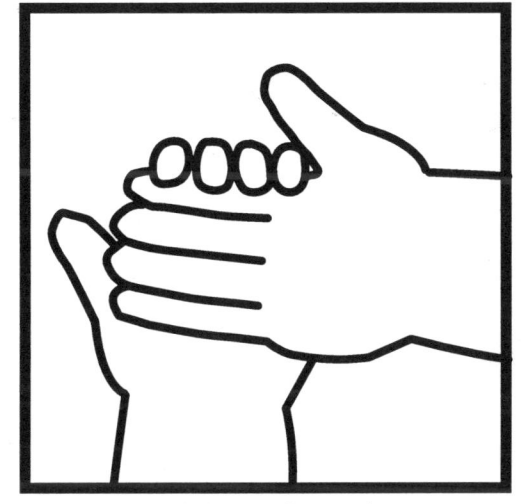

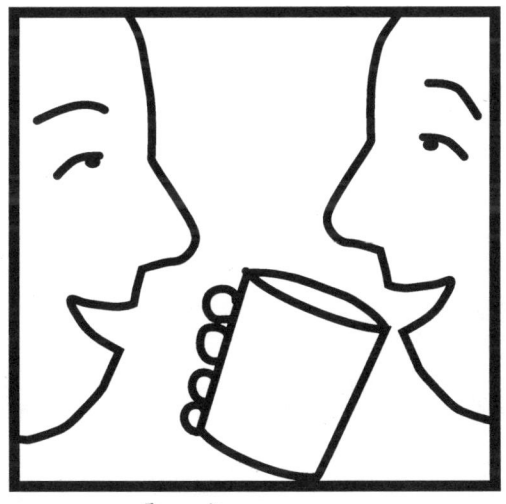

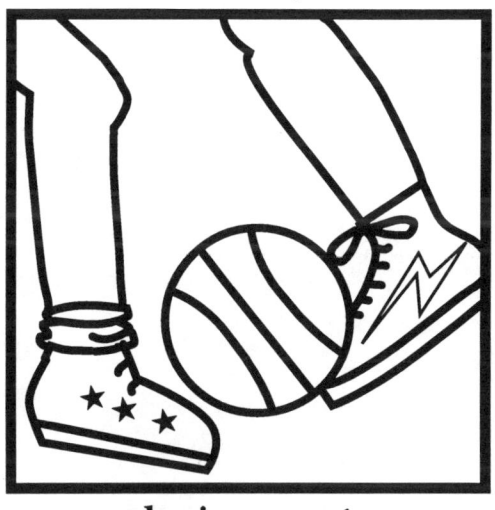

holding hands	kissing
sharing a cup	playing sports
dancing	hugging

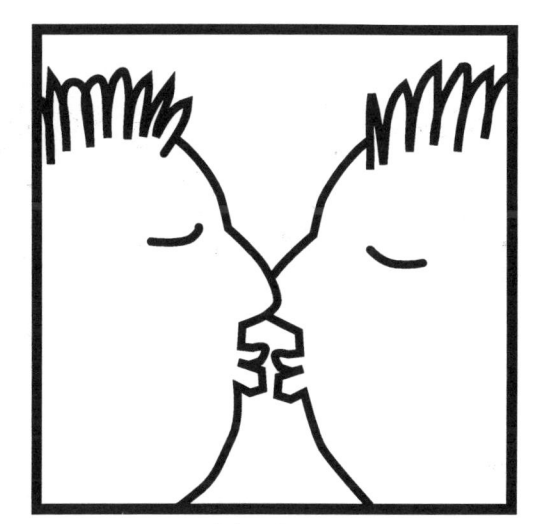

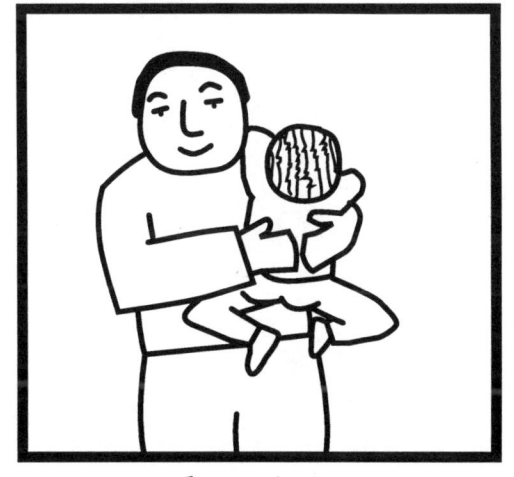

© ETR Associates

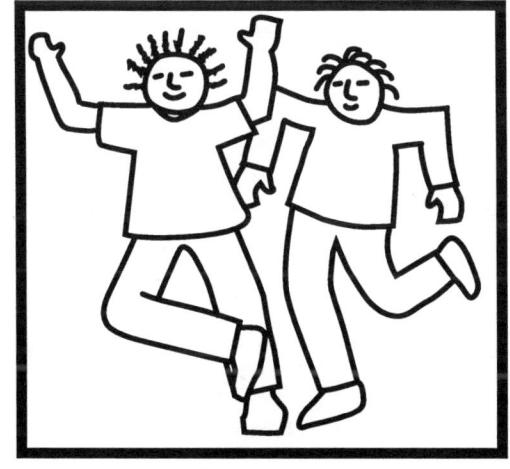

How AIDS Works: Grades K–3

FAMILY ACTIVITY SHEET 4.2

What About AIDS?

Dear Parents,

In Unit 4 of the AIDS curriculum, students are learning why AIDS is hard to pass from one person to another and that children don't have to worry about getting it.

These are the concepts for Unit 4:

1. The AIDS germ is an "inside germ." It is not easily passed from one person to another.

2. The AIDS germ can only be passed from one person to another through a few activities, and most students in elementary school do not do these things. This is why they do not need to worry about having or getting AIDS.

3. The AIDS germ damages the immune system, and this makes it hard for the body to fight off diseases.

Student Work

As part of these lessons, students completed an activity sheet or a drawing. If your child has an activity sheet, ask what it shows. You can also ask questions 1 and 2. If your child has a drawing, ask about the drawing and what it shows. You can also ask questions 3 and 4.

Activity Sheet:

1. Why is AIDS hard to get?

   The AIDS germ is an "inside" germ. It does not pass from person to person the way cold or flu germs do. The skin protects us, and helps keep "inside" germs inside.

2. Do you have any other questions about AIDS?

(continued)

© ETR Associates

How AIDS Works: Grades K–3

FAMILY ACTIVITY SHEET 4.2
continued

Drawing:

3. What does your drawing show?
4. Do you have any other questions about AIDS?

Further Information

You do not need to have all the facts about AIDS to talk about the topic with your child and respond to questions. If you would like further information about the lessons, please feel free to call me at _____.

If you have questions about AIDS, you can call the National AIDS Hotline at 1-800-342-AIDS, or the local AIDS Hotline at _____.
If your child asks you something about AIDS and you do not know the answer, you could call the hotline together for more information.

Sincerely,

_____
(Teacher name)

Unit 5

Preventing AIDS

Time 45 minutes

Unit Objective Students will be able to describe what AIDS does to the immune system and how people can protect themselves from the AIDS germ.

Concepts
1. There are simple steps people can take to protect themselves from AIDS.
2. There are just a few things that are important for children to know to protect themselves from AIDS.

Overview In Unit 4, students learned that the AIDS germ is a special kind of germ and that AIDS is hard to get. They learned what activities transmit the AIDS germ, and understand that these behaviors are not commonly practiced by children their age. This unit expands on some of this information, with further demonstrations about how AIDS affects the body. A presentation explains what steps children and adults can take to protect themselves.

Unit Summary

Activity 1. How Does AIDS Make People Sick? (20 minutes): After a brief *review* of concepts from earlier units, the teacher directs a *roleplay* in which students take on the roles of a healthy person, germs trying to infect that person, and the immune system protecting the person. They then enact the AIDS germ infecting the person and restricting the immune system so it cannot fight off other diseases.

Activity 2. Preventing AIDS (10 minutes): The teacher provides a brief *lecture* about simple precautions people can take to protect themselves from AIDS, and emphasizes that scientists and doctors are working hard to find ways to help people with AIDS.

Evaluation. What Kids Need to Know About AIDS (10–15 minutes): Older students complete a *drawing* to show their understanding of what children need to know about AIDS. Younger students complete an *activity sheet* of picture choices about what to do in situations that might present a risk of blood-to-blood contact.

Family Activity. The *family activity* offers students a chance to discuss the lesson with parents.

Developmental Framework

- Younger students may need considerably more direction and help in the roleplay presented in Activity 1, as well as help understanding what the play symbolizes.

- Younger students may also have less information to volunteer in the discussion section of Activity 2.

- An activity sheet is available as an alternative to the drawing activity in the Evaluation.

- Once again, older students may be able to make the distinction between HIV and AIDS. If students are able to understand this distinction, use the terms appropriately. (HIV is the name of the virus that causes AIDS, and anyone infected with HIV is said to have HIV infection, or HIV. AIDS is a serious disease that develops after people have been infected with HIV for some time.)

Review Teacher Content Summary for Unit 5:

- **Preventing AIDS: Important Concepts for Children** (p. 153)

Get Ready *For Evaluation have:*

- **Staying Safe from AIDS** (Student Activity Sheet 5.1) *(for younger students)*
- drawing materials *(for older students)*
- **Protecting Kids from AIDS** (Family Activity Sheet 5.2) *(for all students)*

Activity 1

How Does AIDS Make People Sick?

Time	20 minutes.
Objective	Students will be able explain how the AIDS germ makes people sick, and how people who have the AIDS germ look and feel.

■ **Note:** Be thoughtful in selecting students to play the roles of a person, the person's immune system, flu and cold germs, and the AIDS germ. For example, students who have had problems being scapegoated by other children might be better off as representatives of the immune system than as germs. Children who have chronic illness themselves or who have family members affected by HIV would also not be a good choice for the AIDS germ because this might give other students the impression that this student actually does carry the AIDS virus.

Review concepts Use the Review Guide (p. 157) to review concepts from earlier units. Areas where students have demonstrated successful understanding of the concepts can be reviewed briefly; review those where concepts may still present a challenge in more depth.

Ask one or more of the questions provided for each previous unit, confirming answers that demonstrate understanding of the concepts and clarifying any misconceptions.

Assign roles to students Explain to students that the lesson will start with a short play presented by several students. The play will explain what the AIDS germ does to the immune system.

(continued)

This activity is based on an activity developed by Donald Leach, a teacher in San Francisco's George Washington High School.

Activity 1 **How Does AIDS Make People Sick?** *continued*

Select volunteers to play the roles in the first part of the play. As you describe the roles and select volunteers, demonstrate the roles so students understand what to do. The roles for the first part of the play include a healthy person, 2 or more people to play cold germs, and a person to play the immune system. For the second part of the play, the roles include the same healthy person, 2 people to play AIDS germs, and 2 or more people to play other kinds of germs.

Introduce the roleplay to students:

> *Is there someone in the class who is feeling very healthy and strong today?* (Select a volunteer.) *Good, you will play the healthy person in our play.*

> *Is there anyone here who has ever had a cold?* (Select 2 volunteers.) *You can play cold germs. Remember, these are germs that can be passed easily between people. You might want to cough a little bit when you get up here.*

> *Is there someone here who likes to protect people, who will stand up for someone who's being hurt?* (Select a volunteer.) *Good, you will play the helper cells.*

Perform first part of roleplay

Help students walk through their roles to perform the first part of the play. (Use students' actual names in the play.)

> *Here is Helen. She is healthy and strong. And over here are Michael and Dinorah. They are germs from someone who has a cold. What can Helen do to keep from getting this cold?*

Look for and confirm responses that describe ways to prevent diseases transmitted by casual contact, such as not sharing cups, not getting too close to someone who is coughing, not touching used tissues.

> *All these things will help Helen protect herself. But sometimes germs like this do get into the body. Then what happens? The helper cells in the person's body start to fight off the germs. Kumi is playing Helen's helper cells. Now, if the cold germs get into Helen's body, her helper cells will fight them off.*

(continued)

How AIDS Works: Grades K–3

Activity 1 How Does AIDS Make People Sick? *continued*

Have the "germs" try to get close to Helen, and have her "helper cells" push them away.

These helper cells are strong and healthy!

Perform second part of roleplay Select volunteers for the second part of the play. Again, describe the roles as you select the players.

Does someone else want to help us with the play? We need a couple of people who can pretend to be AIDS germs. (Select 2 volunteers.) And are there a couple more people who could play some other kind of germ? (Select 2 or 3 volunteers.) Good, you come up and play other germs.

Again, help students walk through their roles to perform the second part of the play.

Now, imagine that some AIDS germs got into Helen's healthy body. Remember, we are just doing this play as a demonstration. Children do not usually get AIDS, especially children your age.

What do you suppose those AIDS germs are going to do? They are going to attack the helper cells! They will make it impossible for the helper cells to fight off other germs.

Have the "AIDS germ" students restrain the "helper cell's" arms, so that this student can no longer push away the other "germs." Have all the "germs" come up and touch Helen.

Now, when other kinds of germs get into the body, what happens? You can see that the helper cells can no longer fight them off.

Thank all the players and lead a round of applause for them.

Activity 1 How Does AIDS Make People Sick? *continued*

Discuss how AIDS makes people sick

Explain the following facts to students:

- The body has millions of helper cells and makes more of them all the time. But, after many years, the AIDS germ finally causes the number of helper cells to drop. Until then, the person will usually feel healthy.

- People with the AIDS germ in their body often feel and look healthy for 5 or 10 years, or even more. You cannot tell just by looking at someone whether he or she has the AIDS germ.

- When people with the AIDS germ do get sick, there is no single way they look. Some people will look completely normal. Some people might look very tired, become very thin or have difficulty walking. Others might have trouble breathing, get bruises easily or have terrible headaches. These are all symptoms of other diseases, too. You cannot tell just by looking at someone whether he or she has the AIDS germ, even if the person looks very sick.

Ongoing Assessment

Use the following questions to assess whether students understand that the AIDS germ damages helper cells so the body is unable to fight off other germs, and that there is no specific way a person with the AIDS germ looks or feels.

- What happens to the helper cells when the AIDS germ gets inside a person's body?

   The cells are damaged and cannot fight germs. When other germs invade the body, the helper cells cannot fight them off, and the person gets sick.

- What does a person who has the AIDS germ inside his or her body look like?

   People with the AIDS germ can look all kinds of ways; some people look very sick, but some people look and feel healthy.

How AIDS Works: Grades K–3

Activity 2

Preventing AIDS

Time	10 minutes.
Objective	Students will be able to describe ways people can protect themselves from infection with the AIDS germ.
Teacher Background	• Preventing AIDS: Important Concepts for Children (p. 153)

Review how the AIDS germ is passed

Remind students of the ways the AIDS germ is passed from person to person.

- Blood-to-blood contact
- Mother-to-baby transmission
- Close sexual contact
- Sharing needles for taking drugs

Also remind students that very few young children get AIDS. Young children who have the AIDS germ probably got it before they were born. They did not get it from playing with another child or being around someone who has the AIDS germ. If students know people who have the AIDS germ in their bodies, students do not need to be afraid to be around them or play with them.

Describe ways to avoid AIDS

Ask students to think about ways people can be sure they do not get AIDS. Emphasize that this is an especially important question for teenagers and adults, since they are the people most likely to do the things that expose people to the AIDS germ.

Look for opportunities to confirm or explain the following:

- Don't use drugs. (Clarification: don't share *injection needles* for taking drugs.)

(continued)

Activity 2   Preventing AIDS, *continued*

- Avoid all kinds of blood-to-blood contact (sharing any kind of needle, touching someone else's blood, sharing razors).
- Don't have sex.
- Don't touch or pick up used drug needles.
- If a person doesn't have sex with anyone and does not take drugs using injection needles, he or she doesn't need to worry about getting AIDS.
- We can all live well without using drugs, but most grown-ups do want to have sex sometimes. They know ways to protect themselves from the AIDS germ when they have sex.

Answer any questions, summarize and check students' comprehension.

Ongoing Assessment Use the following question to assess whether students can describe different ways people can protect themselves from infection with the AIDS germ.

■ What are some things people can do to make sure they do not get the AIDS germ?

Don't take drugs with needles. Don't touch anyone else's blood. Don't have sex. Don't share any kind of needle that might have blood on it. Don't touch or pick up used drug needles.

How AIDS Works: Grades K–3

Evaluation

What Kids Need to Know About AIDS

Time	10–15 minutes.
Objective	Students will be able to demonstrate their understanding of ways to prevent AIDS.
Teacher Background	• Preventing AIDS: Important Concepts for Children (p. 153)
Materials	• Staying Safe from AIDS (5.1) OR drawing materials • Protecting Kids from AIDS (5.2)

Discuss what students need to know about AIDS

Based on the information you have covered concerning AIDS, ask students to discuss what children need to know about AIDS.

Use the discussion to emphasize the following points:

- There are just a few things children their age need to know to protect themselves from AIDS.

- Children their age are not usually in danger of getting the AIDS germ.

- They need to use common sense about not touching blood or used injection needles.

- If children come into contact with blood, they should wash the blood off with soap and warm water. Remind them that the skin is an excellent barrier against germs.

- Remind them also that even if they come into contact with someone else's blood, they do not have a risk for AIDS unless that person has the AIDS germ in his or her blood. Most people do not have the AIDS germ in their blood.

- Most children sometimes have questions or worries about AIDS. There are people students can go to if questions about AIDS come up for them in the future. (Identify who some of these people might be—parents, school nurse, teacher.)

Evaluation	**What Kids Need to Know About AIDS,** *continued*

Students complete assignment

For younger students:

Distribute Student Activity Sheet 5.1, **Staying Safe from AIDS**. Ask students to look at the pictures on the activity sheet. Each set of pictures gives students a choice about what to do in a situation. Ask them to circle the correct thing to do.

Go over each situation with students and discuss to check comprehension.

- For the choice presented in the first pair of pictures (finding a used syringe on the ground), ask students which is the better choice: to pick it up or get a grown-up to help? Then ask why getting a grown-up to help is the better choice.

  A child could accidentally get stuck with the needle on a used syringe, and this could be dangerous. A grown-up will be able to pick up the syringe and throw it away in a safe place, where it will not hurt anyone else.

- For the second pair of pictures (helping a child with a bloody nose), emphasize that children should not touch other people's blood and that a grown-up will know how to help the child in the safest way possible.

For older students:

Distribute drawing materials. Ask students to draw a picture showing something children their age need to know about AIDS. Students with writing skills could also write a short essay describing what the picture shows.

You can also include the following instruction to the class:

> *We have learned that close sexual contact is a way of spreading the AIDS germ. For this activity, however, I would prefer that you not draw a picture of how AIDS is spread in this way. I would like you to draw a picture of one of the other things you learned about AIDS.*

Ask students to describe their pictures and confirm that the drawings are consistent with the facts about AIDS discussed in class.

Family Activity

Distribute Family Activity Sheet 5.2, **Protecting Kids from AIDS**. Ask students to take their drawings or activity sheets home and discuss their work with their parents.

How AIDS Works: Grades K–3

STUDENT ACTIVITY SHEET 5.1

Name _____

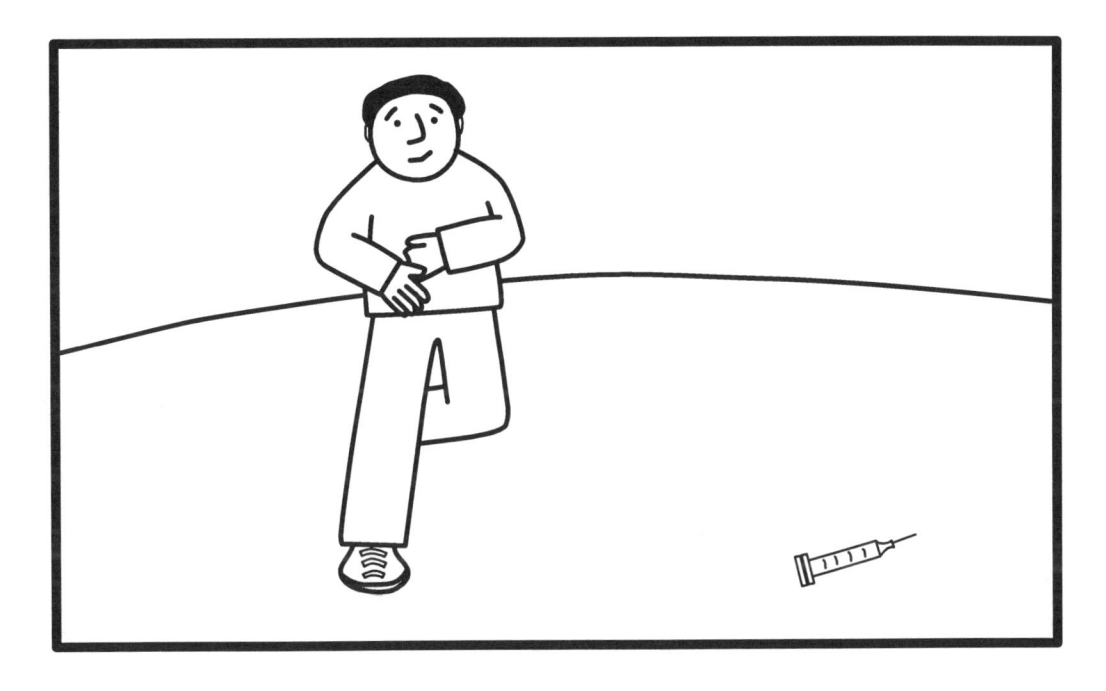

Staying Safe from AIDS

You find a used syringe on the ground. Do you (1) pick it up, or (2) get a grown-up to help?

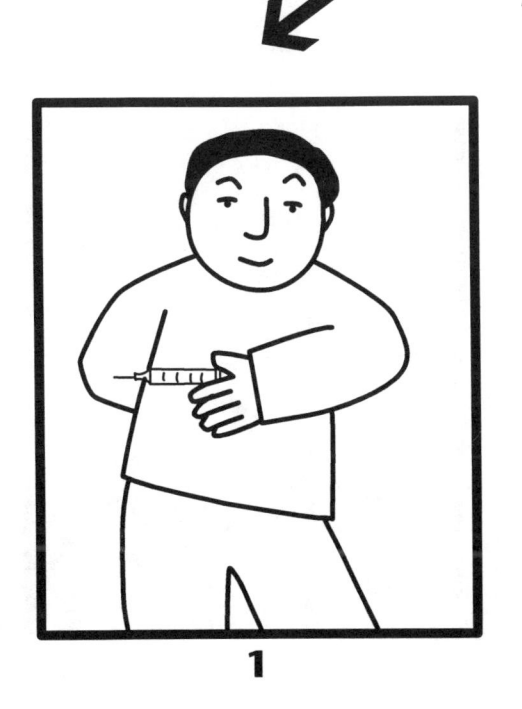

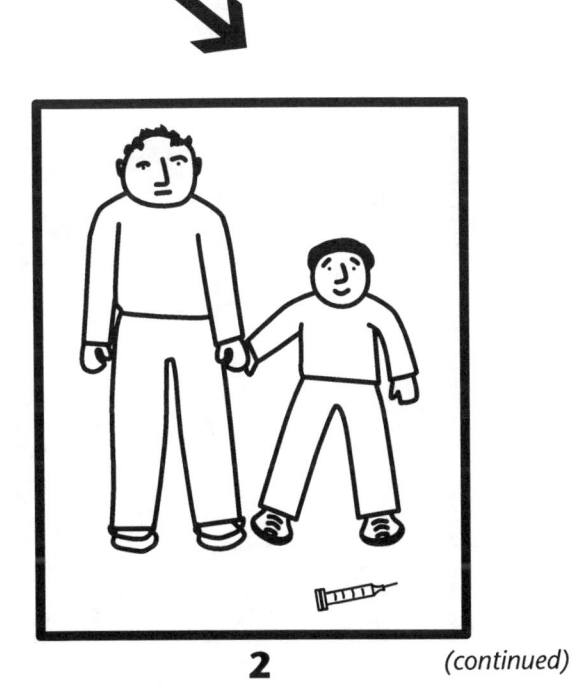

1

2

(continued)

How AIDS Works: Grades K–3

STUDENT ACTIVITY SHEET 5.1
continued

Staying Safe from AIDS

A kid has a bloody nose. Do you
(1) touch the blood, or (2) get a grown-up to help?

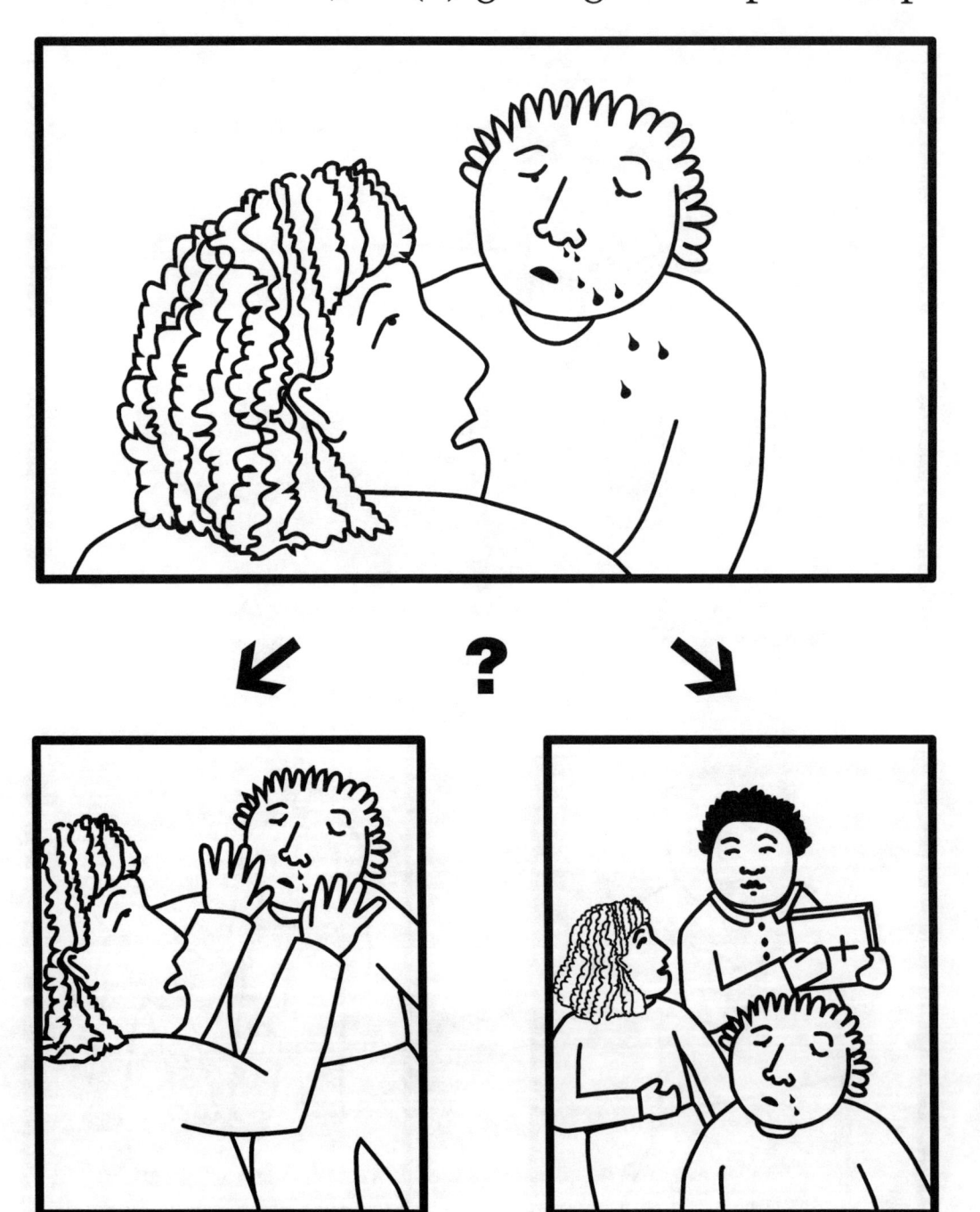

1

2

FAMILY ACTIVITY SHEET 5.2

Protecting Kids from AIDS

Dear Parents,

In Unit 5 of the AIDS curriculum, students are learning what AIDS does to the immune system and how people can protect themselves from the AIDS virus.

These are the concepts for Unit 5:

1. There are simple steps people can take to protect themselves from AIDS.
2. There are just a few things that are important for children to know to protect themselves from AIDS.

Student Work

As part of these lessons, students completed an activity sheet or a drawing. If your child has an activity sheet, ask what it shows. You can also ask questions 1 and 2. If your child has a drawing, ask about the drawing and what it shows. You can also ask questions 3 and 4.

Activity Sheet:

1. What do these pictures show?

   The drawings show 2 situations children might face that could bring them in contact with the AIDS virus or other blood-borne germs. Students were asked to circle the better choice in each situation.

2. Why are these the better choices in each of these situations?

   The better choices are those in which contact with someone else's blood is avoided. For example: Do not touch a used syringe. Do not touch someone else's blood if they are hurt, but get a grown-up to help.

Drawing:

3. What does your drawing show?
4. Why is this important for kids your age to know?

(continued)

How AIDS Works: Grades K–3

FAMILY ACTIVITY SHEET 5.2

continued

Further Information

You do not need to have all the facts about AIDS to talk about the topic with your child and respond to questions. If you would like further information about the lessons, please feel free to call me at _____.

If you have questions about AIDS, you can call the National AIDS Hotline at 1-800-342-AIDS, or the local AIDS Hotline at _____.
If your child asks you something about AIDS and you do not know the answer, you could call the hotline together for more information.

Sincerely,

_____

(Teacher name)

Unit 6

Helping Out

Time 30 minutes, plus time for review and speaker, film or story

Unit Objective Students will be able to describe some of the ways people who are affected by AIDS or other serious illnesses might feel, and be able to suggest ways to help.

Concepts 1. People with AIDS and their families need and deserve support and care.

Overview Children who have a family member or friend with HIV or AIDS often experience additional distress when peers ridicule or demean people with AIDS. Children who have experienced other kinds of serious illness or disability in their families have also heard taunts, blame or simple insensitivity. Unit 6 includes activities that address support for people with AIDS and their families.

These activities help young children build a compassionate and sympathetic perspective towards people with serious illnesses and provide an opportunity for closure to the curriculum. This unit gives students something practical they can do to help—a reassuring step for children in building an understanding of this serious and sometimes frightening disease.

Unit 6 also gives you an opportunity to review selected concepts from earlier units. Choose areas of focus based on what you feel would be most useful for your students. You could focus on a topic

(continued)

that was particularly interesting to the class, or go over something that did not really seem clear to students. Any unanswered questions raised during the lessons can be addressed.

You could also invite a guest speaker, show a film or read a story. Suggested procedures for these kinds of activities are included in the Teacher Content Summary for Unit 6 (p. 155).

Unit Summary   **Activity 1: Curriculum Review (time varies):** The teacher *reviews* areas covered by the curriculum.

Activity 2: Guest Speaker, Film or Story (time varies): The teacher invites a *guest speaker* to address the class; shows a *film* and discusses it with students; or reads a *story* and discusses it with students.

Activity 3: Caring About People with AIDS and Their Families (10–15 minutes): A series of *discussion questions* invites students to think about what it might be like to have a friend or family member with the AIDS germ and what steps people can take to help.

Activity 4: Making Cards (15 minutes): Students *make cards* for people with AIDS or other serious illnesses that can be delivered to a local hospital or nursing facility.

Family Activity. The *family activity* offers students a chance to discuss the lesson with parents.

Developmental Framework
- Younger students may have less information to volunteer in the discussion during Activity 3.
- For children who are less comfortable or capable with drawing and card making in Activity 4, you can provide a photocopied card with space for students to color and/or sign their names.

Terms to Use
- kindness
- compassion

Review   Teacher Content Summary for Unit 6:
- **Guest Speakers, Videos and Stories** (p. 155)

Get Ready   *For Activity 2 have:*

- guest speaker, OR
- film and discussion questions, OR
- story and discussion questions

For Activity 4 have:

- crayons and scissors
- **Sorry You Don't Feel Well** (Student Activity Sheet 6.1) *(for younger students)*
- drawing materials *(for older students)*
- **Helping Out** (Family Activity Sheet 6.2) *(for all students)*

Activity 1

Curriculum Review

> Time   Varies
> Objective   Students will demonstrate learning of concepts from earlier units.

Review concepts Use the Review Guide (p. 157) to review concepts from earlier units. Areas where students have demonstrated successful understanding of the concepts can be reviewed briefly; review those where concepts may still present a challenge in more depth.

Ask one or more of the questions provided for each unit, confirming answers that demonstrate understanding of the concepts and clarifying any misconceptions.

Activity 2

Guest Speaker, Film or Story

Time	Varies
Objective	Students will have an opportunity to think or learn about AIDS through a special resource, such as a speaker, film or story.
Teacher Background	• Guest Speakers, Videos and Stories (p. 155)

Introduce guest speaker, film or story

Announce to the class that today they will hear a speaker (see a film, read a story) that will help them think and learn more about AIDS. Introduce the speaker, or announce the name of the film or story. Have the speaker make his or her presentation to the class, or show the film or read the story to students.

Discuss the presentation

Allow students to ask any questions they may have for the speaker or about the film or story. Keep the discussion focused on the important points of the presentation, and clarify any new information that may have been presented to be sure students understand it. Thank the guest speaker.

Activity 3

Caring About People with AIDS and Their Families

Time	10–15 minutes
Objective	Students will identify and discuss kindness and acceptance as important features of caring for people with AIDS or other serious illnesses.

Introduce activity

Acknowledge that much of the focus of these lessons about health and AIDS has been on the way things work—how germs make people sick, what people can do to stay healthy, and what the AIDS germ does to the immune system.

Now, you are going to talk about feelings. The class will think about how people feel when they, or someone in their family, has the AIDS germ.

■ **Note:** The primary goal is to help students think about the emotional effects of AIDS on individuals and families. However, as you gather responses, you can also confirm or clarify information about HIV and AIDS as the need arises.

Discuss emotional effects of AIDS

Ask one or more of the following questions, depending on students' interest and experience.

- Has anyone in this class seen movies, television programs or news reports showing people who have the AIDS germ?

  If possible, help students identify someone they know of who has the AIDS virus. This might be a celebrity, a character in a recent movie, or someone in a story or video shown to the class. The idea is to personalize the disease by giving it a human face.

(continued)

Activity 3   Caring About People with AIDS and Their Families, continued

- What do you suppose life is like for people who have the AIDS germ?

  Validate responses that talk about people feeling uncomfortable physically, but try to direct the discussion towards people's emotional states.

- How do you think people feel if a member of their family has the AIDS germ?

  Validate students' responses. People may feel sad, angry or scared.

- Some people with AIDS have been treated badly by others. Have any of you heard of these kinds of things happening?

  If students do not volunteer some examples, you may want to offer some descriptions. Examples: Someone being fired from a job for having AIDS; someone saying mean things to a person with AIDS, or teasing him or her for being sick; someone refusing to serve a person with AIDS in a restaurant.

- Why do you suppose these kinds of things happen?

  People don't understand about AIDS. People have wrong information about AIDS. People might be afraid. Some people just aren't very nice. Look for these or other responses that are appropriate.

- How do you think that person, or members of his or her family, have felt when these things have happened?

  Validate students' responses.

- Earlier in this class, we talked about ways you have been helped when you were feeling sick. What kind of help can people offer to someone they know with AIDS?

  Be nice to them. Make them cards. Be a good friend. Visit them. Don't be afraid of them. Look for these or other responses that are appropriate.

- What kind of help can people offer to someone with a different kind of serious illness—cancer, perhaps, or heart disease?

  Look for and confirm responses that suggest many of the same kinds of things are helpful to anyone with any kind of serious illness.

How AIDS Works: Grades K–3

Activity 3 Caring About People with AIDS and Their Families, *continued*

Summarize discussion Summarize and conclude the discussion. If possible, based on what students have offered, emphasize the importance of kindness and compassion for people with all kinds of serious illnesses, including AIDS.

Ongoing Assessment Use the following question to assess whether students can demonstrate a sense of concern and acceptance for people with AIDS or other serious illnesses.

- What kinds of things can we do to help people with AIDS or other serious illnesses?

    Be a friend. Don't be mean to them. Let them know you like them. Visit them. Help them out if you can.

Activity 4

Making Cards

Time	15 minutes.
Objective	Students will put into practice their conclusions about kindness and acceptance for people with AIDS or other serious illnesses by making cards for them.
Materials	• crayons and scissors • Sorry You Don't Feel Well (6.1) OR drawing materials • Helping Out (6.2)

■ **Note:** Before doing this activity, identify a hospital, hospice or nursing facility serving people with AIDS or other serious illnesses that would like to receive cards from your students. Some helpful people to contact to make these arrangements include the Director of Volunteer Services, the Public Relations office, or, in smaller facilities, the Executive Director's office. You might ask your contact person what messages would be most appreciated by the facility's patients, and share that information with your students when they are planning their cards.

Introduce activity Remind students of the importance of showing kindness and acceptance for people with the AIDS germ.

Let them know that now they will have a chance to put this into practice, by making cards for people who have AIDS (or some other serious illness).

Describe card recipients Describe the people who are going to receive the cards. This might include what facility they are in, what kinds of physical problems they are dealing with, and what it will be like for them to receive cards that let them know people are thinking about them.

If the cards are not going to people with AIDS or HIV, be sure students understand this. You do not want cards that say, "Sorry you

(continued)

How AIDS Works: Grades K–3 **125**

Activity 4   **Making Cards,** *continued*

---

have AIDS," if the cards are actually going to people with other types of illnesses.

Students make cards

For younger students:

Distribute Student Activity Sheet 6.1, **Sorry You Don't Feel Well**, and crayons and scissors. Show students how to cut out and fold the card. Help students cut out the card if necessary.

Ask students to color the front of the card, sign their names inside, and add further drawings if they wish.

For older students:

Distribute drawing materials. Ask students to make a card and sign it. Students with writing skills could add a message to the recipient of the card. As a group, discuss briefly what kinds of messages would be most appreciated by the recipients of the cards.

Students share cards

If time and class size allow, invite students to say something about the card they drew and what it means to them.

Collect cards

Collect the cards and arrange to have them delivered to the facility. If possible, gather some feedback from your contact person to share with students after the cards have been received.

Family Activity

Distribute Family Activity Sheet 6.2, **Helping Out**. Ask students to take the activity sheet home and discuss the questions on it with their parents.

STUDENT ACTIVITY SHEET 6.1

Name _____

Sorry You Don't Feel Well

Sorry You Don't Feel Well

fold

© ETR Associates

How AIDS Works: Grades K–3

127

FAMILY ACTIVITY SHEET 6.2

Helping Out

Dear Parents,

In Unit 6 of the AIDS curriculum, students talked about some of the ways people who are affected by AIDS or other serious illnesses might feel and suggested ways to help.

This is the concept for Unit 6:

1. People with AIDS and their families need and deserve support and care.

Student Work

The AIDS curriculum your child has participated in is now completed. The final unit explored ways to help out people with AIDS or other serious illnesses. Please help your child review the lessons by talking about these questions.

1. What are some important things you learned about AIDS?
2. What do you think is the most important thing for children to know about AIDS?
3. If you had a good friend or someone in the family who had a serious illness, what would you want to do to help that person out?

You may want to take this opportunity to talk over your family's experiences with friends or relatives who have had serious illnesses. You could remind your child of the experience, ask how he or she feels about it now, and check to see if your child has any questions about what happened or how people helped out.

(continued)

How AIDS Works: Grades K–3

FAMILY ACTIVITY SHEET 6.2
continued

Further Information

Your child may continue to have questions about AIDS. Remember, you do not need to have all the facts about AIDS to talk about the topic with your child and respond to questions. If you have future questions about AIDS, you can call the National AIDS Hotline at 1-800-342-AIDS, or the local AIDS Hotline at _____.

If you have any comments or suggestions about the AIDS curriculum, please feel free to call me at _____.

Sincerely,

_____
(Teacher name)

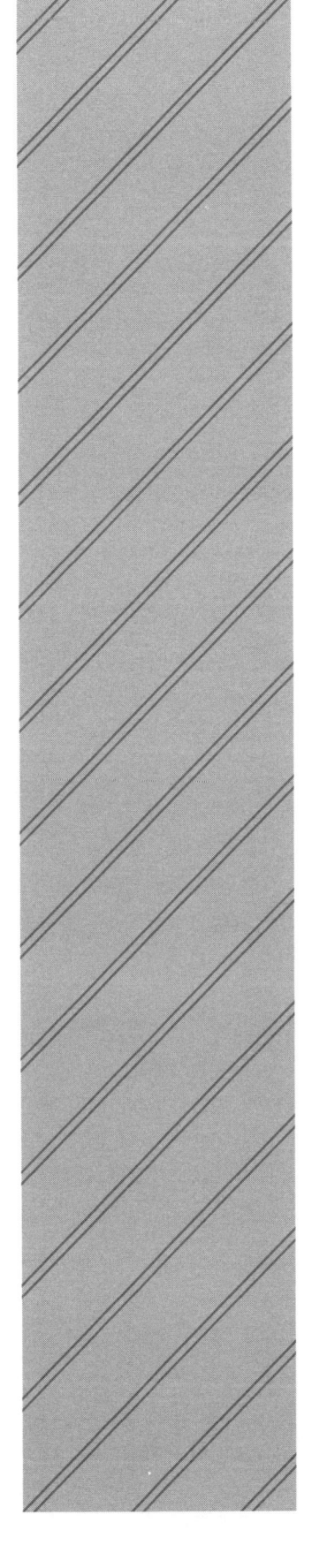

For the Teacher

A Resource Section

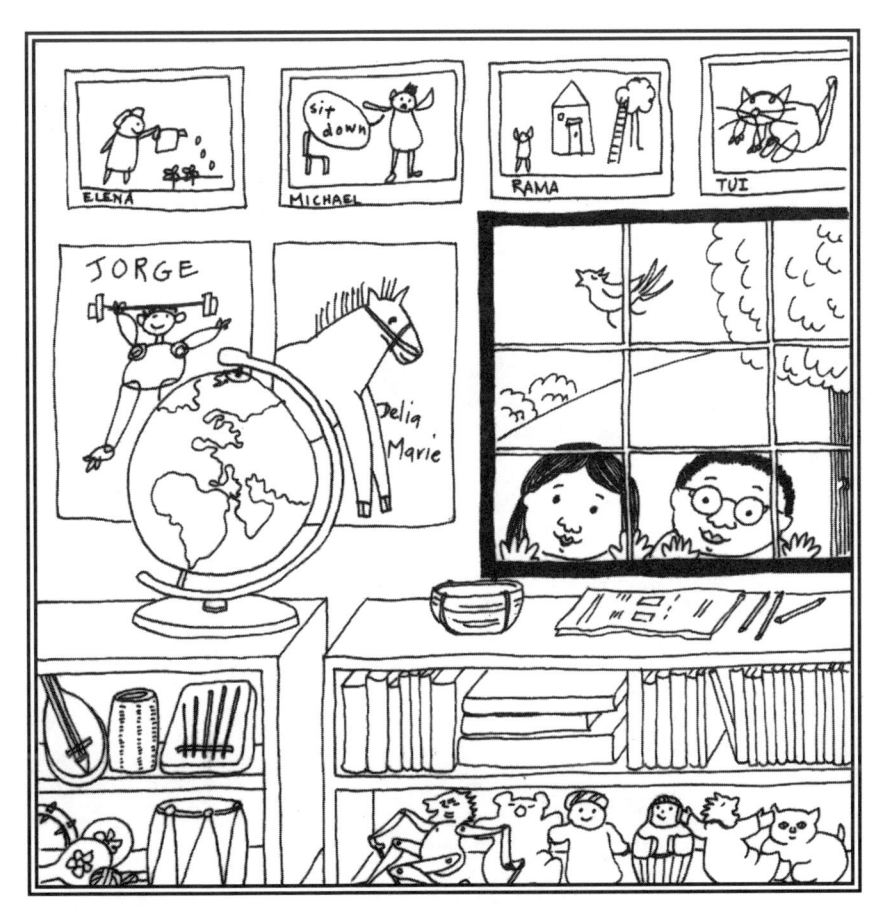

Teacher Content Summaries

Unit 1
Helping Young Children Understand How Illnesses Are Different

WHEN ADULTS ARE FACED with something they do not understand, they often think back to prior experience. Then they make inferences about this new situation based on what they learned in the past. Adults have many years of practice drawing conclusions about new situations by generalizing this way from earlier knowledge and experience.

Know that Children Overgeneralize

Children, faced with new ideas or information, do the same thing. They look to past experience and knowledge to develop a better understanding of new situations or information. They do not, however, have the same wealth of experience to draw from as adults, nor do they have the ability to think about situations at the same level of abstraction. Children *overgeneralize* from previous experience to current experience, and thus often make errors in the conclusions they draw.

Teachers of young children often see this process at work. A child who is baffled by the new task of multiplication completes the arithmetic problems by adding rather than multiplying the figures. A student who learns in science class that male songbirds are the ones who sing states that science has proven boys can sing better than girls. And a child who has heard repeatedly that colds and flus are easily spread by coughs and sharing cups believes that AIDS can also be transmitted in this manner.

Children must learn how to differentiate among illnesses before information about AIDS and HIV can truly be useful to them. Without this ability, they will make the leaps of understanding that follow from overgeneralization. Examples of this can be seen in the mistaken ideas children may develop about AIDS from television and peers: AIDS is caused by drugs, so people who smoke cigarettes may get AIDS. Dirty needles spread AIDS, there is dirt on the playground, germs live in dirt, so maybe the AIDS germ lives in dirt and the playground can give people AIDS. People get AIDS from sleeping together, so a child who shares a bed with a sibling might get AIDS.

How AIDS Works: Grades K–3

Unit 1, *continued*

For adults, the straightforward juxtaposition of different facts may make distinctions self-evident. This technique does *not* work with young children. Imagine an adult who understands that diseases caused by bacteria can usually be cured with antibiotics, but that antibiotics do not improve viral illnesses. She is told she has a bacterial disease and asks if an antibiotic is available. At another time, diagnosed with a viral flu, she does not ask for an antibiotic. The distinctions between a bacterial and viral illness are evident to her.

A young child, however, learns that AIDS is caused by a virus, and that the body cannot fight off this virus. He also hears there is no cure for AIDS and that people usually die of the disease. When he later develops a cold, his mother tells him it is caused by a virus, and the best "cure" is for him to rest and let his body heal itself. He worries that his body will be unable to fight off this virus, and that he may die. The distinctions between the AIDS virus and his cold virus are not evident to him.

Emphasize Broader Concepts

Children learn to differentiate between illnesses not by studying facts about different illnesses, but by building an understanding of broader conceptual principles: that different illnesses have different causes, different symptoms and different treatments. We also want them to understand that while there are some general things we can state about illnesses as a whole, there are also unique aspects to each illness.

This curriculum begins by emphasizing these broader concepts, and then presents facts that further reinforce the concepts. For example, the early lessons stress that different illnesses are spread in different ways. Students' pre-existing knowledge about familiar illnesses is then placed into this conceptual framework.

Later, the curriculum introduces the fact that the AIDS germ, which lives mainly in blood and certain body fluids, is spread through the transfer of infected blood and these other body fluids. It is not spread through the same kinds of behaviors that spread a cold germ, which lives in saliva. Children will be better prepared to learn the unique characteristics of the causes, treatment and prevention of AIDS once they understand that *all* illnesses have unique characteristics.

Children will not learn to differentiate effectively after a single lesson on these concepts. They will need to have the concepts repeated, with frequent reinforcement through examples and explanations. For this reason, review segments are built into each unit.

Help Children Learn to Differentiate

In addition, look for student comments and discussion that demonstrate the ability to differentiate. Whenever possible, emphasize the 3 important areas of difference between illnesses—causes, symptoms and treatments. Take discussions beyond the juxtaposition of facts, to help children learn how to differentiate.

Unit 1, *continued*

For example, you might ask the class, "Can you get AIDS by sharing a spoon with someone who has AIDS?" Your students, properly tutored, answer, "No." Many teachers would stop here, praising the students for their correct answer. However, a teacher exploring the children's ability to differentiate between illnesses would look for more than the parroting back of facts. "No, you can't get AIDS from sharing a spoon, " the teacher confirms. "But what kind of illness *could* you get this way?"

"Where are germs found?" asks a teacher. "Germs are found *everywhere*!" exclaim the students. "Yes," says the teacher, "but is every kind of germ found everywhere?" This kind of question reminds students that they have learned that some germs, like the AIDS germ, live in only a few places.

These kinds of questions encourage students to think back to other experience and knowledge, and give them the opportunity to understand and express contrasts between that knowledge and new information. With repeated practice at this skill, children will be able to apply these principles more often and more effectively, not only in terms of knowledge about AIDS, but in other domains as well.

Communicable and Non-Communicable Illnesses

YOUNG CHILDREN ARE CAPABLE of understanding the basic concepts of communicable disease—most important, that under the appropriate circumstances, one person carrying a disease-causing germ can pass that germ on to another person. Giving young children the tools they need to master concepts about communicable and non-communicable illnesses can help them develop a better understanding about AIDS. Additionally, and of equal importance, we build their future capacity to understand and respond to all kinds of communicable illnesses.

This summary reviews important general concepts about communicable and non-communicable diseases and gives background information on a number of common illnesses that may arise as topics of discussion in the curriculum. Your class may not need information as detailed as what follows. But being familiar with these concepts can help you approach the lessons with greater confidence.

General Concepts About Disease

Some illnesses are caused by germs that are passed from person to person. These are called "communicable" diseases. The easiest way to explain this to children is to explain "there are some sicknesses you can catch from someone, and some sicknesses you can't catch from someone."

A communicable disease can only be passed from one person to another under the following circumstances:

How AIDS Works: Grades K–3

Unit 1, *continued*

The first person must have the disease.

The disease must be infectious. That is, the disease-causing organism, or *pathogen*, must be in a form capable of causing infection in someone else.

In some cases, a person may be most infectious at the earliest stages of an illness, before any symptoms are present. For example, children with chicken pox are most contagious 1 or 2 days *before* (and shortly after) the rash appears. This is why chicken pox spreads rapidly through a school even if care is taken to keep all children known to be affected out of the school until they are no longer contagious.

The pathogen must enter the body of the second person. Different pathogens enter the body in different ways. For example, viruses that cause the common cold are spread by close person-to-person contact, through the air in small droplets of mucus or saliva (respiratory droplets) that enter the air when an infected individual coughs or sneezes, or by touching objects (called "fomites") that are contaminated with infected mucus or saliva.

The virus that causes Hepatitis A is passed through fecal material, which is one reason it is important for people to wash their hands well after using the bathroom. The virus that causes AIDS can be passed through infected blood, semen or vaginal secretions. The virus that causes pink eye (viral conjunctivitis) is spread by germs in tears. If a boy with pink eye touches his eyes with his hand, then touches another child's hand, and that second child touches her eye, all in a fairly short time period, the second child might get pink eye.

The pathogen must overwhelm the body's initial defenses, enter cells or tissue, reproduce and cause infection. Our bodies are exposed to thousands of pathogens every day. A healthy immune system is so sophisticated that it is able to eradicate most pathogens before they establish infection. Occasionally, however, the system is overwhelmed by the pathogen and disease develops.

In this unit, you will be explaining in simple terms the distinction between illnesses that are communicable and those that are not. Although your class will not need to review at this level of detail, it may be useful to review the following list of common diseases, their causes and symptoms, means of transmission and strategies for preventions.

Communicable Diseases

Colds

Cause: A variety of viruses. There are hundreds of different viruses that cause the common cold. This is why people can catch a cold many different times—each new cold is caused by a virus different from those that have caused illness in the individual in the past.

Symptoms: Fever, headache, congestion, cough, runny nose, sore throat.

Transmission:

- Direct contact with an infected person.

Unit 1, *continued*

- Through small droplets of mucus or saliva (respiratory droplets) that enter the air when an infected individual coughs or sneezes.
- Touching objects (called "fomites") that are contaminated with infected mucus or saliva.

Prevention:

- Persons with colds covering the mouth and nose when sneezing or coughing, and then washing their hands.
- Persons with colds throwing out their own used tissues.
- Washing hands before eating.
- Not sharing eating utensils or cups.

Chicken Pox

Cause: A virus.

Symptoms: Itchy, blister-like rash covers most of the body (the rash will later scab over before healing); mild fever.
People become sick 10–21 days after exposure. In other words, the *incubation period* ranges from 10–21 days.

Transmission:

- Direct contact with an infected person.
- Through small droplets of mucus or saliva (respiratory droplets) that enter the air when an infected individual coughs or sneezes.
- Highly contagious.
- People are contagious 1–2 days before the onset of the rash, and shortly after the onset of the rash.

Prevention: Avoid direct contact with infected person during the contagious period.

Additional notes: Once a person has had chicken pox, he or she usually will not catch it again—that is, a lifelong immunity is established. A vaccine is now available as well.

Flu (influenza)

Cause: A variety of viruses.

Symptoms: Fever, headache, muscle aches, sore throat, stuffy nose, cough.

Transmission:

- Direct contact with an infected person.
- Through small droplets of mucus or saliva (respiratory droplets) that enter the air when an infected individual coughs or sneezes.

Prevention: Same as strategies for preventing colds. A vaccine is now available for protection against some strains of influenza.

Measles

Cause: A virus.

Symptoms: Cough, runny nose, red eyes, fever, red bumpy-blotchy rash.

Transmission:

- Direct contact with the mucus or saliva of an infected person.
- Through small droplets of mucus or saliva (respiratory droplets) that enter the air when an infected individual coughs or sneezes.

Prevention: Children are vaccinated against measles beginning at 12–15 months of age, so the disease is now uncommon in the United States.

Unit 1, *continued*

Pink Eye (Viral Conjunctivitis)
Cause: A virus.

Symptoms: White of the eye and inside of the eyelids become red; there may be increased tearing or a clear discharge from the eye(s); cold symptoms, including fever, may be present.

Transmission: Direct contact with tears or discharge from the eye of someone with pink eye, and later contact with one's own eye. (For example, a person with pink eye touches his eye, then shakes someone else's hand, and the second person touches her eye.)

Prevention:

- The person with pink eye avoids touching other people, and washes hands after touching eyes.
- Avoid direct contact with tears or discharge from person with the illness; avoid touching the person; wash hands after any contact.

Additional Note: Bacterial infections, eye irritation, allergies and other conditions may also cause the eye to appear pink or lead to increased tearing or eye discharge.

Infectious Diarrhea
Cause: Bacteria, viruses or parasites.

Symptoms: Diarrhea. May also involve vomiting or fever.

Transmission: Most infectious diarrheas are spread by contact with infected fecal material.

Prevention: Good handwashing, especially after using the bathroom.

Strep Throat
Cause: A particular bacterium, *streptococcus*.

Symptoms: Very painful throat, fever, swollen glands. Very red throat. Pus may be visible on the tonsils. If a red, sandpaper rash also develops, the person is said to have scarlet fever.

Transmission:

- Direct contact with an infected person.
- Through small droplets of mucus or saliva (respiratory droplets) that enter the air when an infected individual coughs or sneezes.

Prevention: Same as strategies for preventing colds.

Tuberculosis (TB)
Cause: Mycobacterium.

Symptoms: Most people with TB will have no symptoms, but will have a positive skin test (a diagnostic tool to detect TB). Those with symptoms may have persistent cough, rapid and heavy breathing, swollen glands, fever, tiredness, weakness, night sweats, weight loss and poor growth.

Transmission: Through small droplets of sputum (respiratory droplets) that enter the air when an infected individual coughs.

Prevention:

- Aggressive treatment of people with active infection (to avoid the spread of the disease to others).

- Avoiding close contact with an infected person.

Additional notes: In the United States, TB is rare in otherwise healthy children.

Non-Communicable Diseases

Appendicitis

Description: An inflammation of the appendix. The appendix is a narrow tube, about 3–4 inches in length, that extends from the blind pouch where the large intestine begins (called the cecum). In acute appendicitis, people usually experience crampy abdominal pain and vomiting, followed by fever and severe pain in the lower right-hand portion of the abdomen. This is where the appendix is found in most people. Surgical removal of the appendix is usually necessary in acute appendicitis.

Cause: Usually due to bacterial infection, which may be started by an obstruction of the appendix.

Asthma

Description: A chronic illness that results in recurrent episodes of breathing difficulty, with shortness of breath, coughing and/or wheezing (a high-pitched whistling noise that comes from the chest, especially when the person breathes out). Asthma attacks (episodes of breathing difficulty) may be triggered by viral respiratory infections (colds), exercise, inhaling cold air, air pollution and allergens (such as pollen).

Cause: Caused by periodic narrowing of the small airways in the lungs, due to spasm of the muscles lining the airways and increased production of mucus in the airways.

Additional notes: People may inherit a tendency to develop asthma (it "runs in families"), but cannot catch it from another person. People who do not have asthma may have a single episode of wheezing with a respiratory infection (such as bronchiolitis or viral pneumonia), whereas those with asthma will have recurrent episodes.

Cancer

Description: A disease characterized by uncontrolled cell growth, with either local growth that develops into a tumor and invades normal tissue, or distant spread (called "metastasis") of cancer cells to other organs or parts of the body, where tumors then develop.

There are many forms of cancer, depending on what type of cell is affected. For example, leukemia (from the Greek *leukos*, meaning "white") is a cancer involving white blood cells.

Cause: The cause of cancer is not clearly determined. However, a few kinds of cancers may be triggered by viral infections, others by exposure to environmental agents (tobacco smoke, asbestos), and others by inherited tendencies.

Important note: Although some kinds of cancers may be triggered by underlying viral infections, the cancer itself is non-communicable. It cannot be spread from one person to another. For the purposes

Unit 1, *continued*

of this lesson, you want students to understand that they do not need to take any special precautions to protect themselves from cancer if they visit or live with someone who has the disease.

Heart Attack

Description: An episode where insufficient blood is supplied to an area of the heart muscle, causing the tissue to die. This causes weakening of the heart muscle and may compromise the heart's ability to pump blood effectively. In severe heart attacks, the heart may stop beating entirely. The medical term for a heart attack is *myocardial infarction* (M.I.).

Cause: Heart attacks are usually caused by a blockage of one of the coronary arteries. These are the arteries that provide blood supply to the heart muscle itself. The blockage is caused by the build-up of fatty substances within the coronary arteries (called *atherosclerosis*). This condition is more common in adults than children. It may be more severe in people with an inherited tendency towards atherosclerosis, or with sedentary lifestyles and high-fat diets.

Poison Ivy (Poison Oak, Poison Sumac)

Description: A red, bumpy rash that often involves itchiness and may exude fluid.

Cause: The skin is irritated by contact with the oil contained on the leaf, stem or root of the plant. Once the oil is washed away (including from clothing), further spread will not occur, even from the fluid exuding from the rash.

Additional notes: The rash often appears about 48 hours after exposure, and areas that were exposed to less of the oil may not develop the rash until a later time. This may make it appear that the rash is "spreading." However, no germ is involved in poison ivy. It cannot be spread from one person to another unless some of the oil still remains on the clothing or body of the first person. This does not meet the criteria for a communicable disease.

Sickle Cell Disease

Description: The red blood cells "sickle" (assume a crescent shape) under certain conditions, causing pain episodes and susceptibility to severe cases of bacterial infections.

Cause: Sickle cell disease is an inherited condition.

Other Diseases

Sexually Transmitted Disease (STD)

If students bring up sexually transmitted diseases (such as syphilis, gonorrhea or HIV), you can certainly use these examples in the activity. You may need to jump ahead and present concepts from Unit 4, however, by making a distinction between diseases that are "easy-to-transmit" and those that are "hard-to-transmit."

"Easy-to-transmit" diseases include those that can be transmitted through air, mucus, droplets of saliva or touching. Explain to students that sexually transmitted diseases are only transmitted under

Unit 1, *continued*

very specific circumstances, not through coughing, shaking hands or sharing cups. You want to avoid giving the impression that someone could catch a sexually transmitted disease simply by visiting someone who has one.

Chronic Illnesses

Some illnesses are *chronic,* or ongoing. Chronic illnesses span the range from mild to severe and disabling or even life-threatening. Some chronic illnesses can be treated, but few can be cured. Sometimes different people with the same chronic illness have very different presentations. One person may be profoundly disabled, while another is barely affected at all.

Examples of chronic illnesses include diabetes, asthma, lupus, rheumatoid arthritis, multiple sclerosis, some types of cancer, Alzheimer's disease and Parkinson's disease. There are many others. HIV disease, because it is a lifelong condition without a cure, is also a chronic illness.

Unusual or Rare Conditions

Children may also mention unusual or rare conditions you are not familiar with. If you know whether or not a disease is communicable, share this with the class. However, don't be afraid to admit you do not know much about a condition. You can always get back to the class later, after you have had some time to do more research or talk to the school nurse or another medical consultant.

Unit 2
Germs and Germ Theory

THIS SUMMARY OFFERS SUGGESTIONS for describing some of the important elements of germ theory in simple terms and straightforward language that is easy for children to understand.

What is a germ?

A germ is a special kind of living thing. It is so small people cannot see it.

There are many different kinds of germs. Some germs can cause sickness if they get inside a person's body.

But not all germs are bad or harmful. Some germs are helpful germs. For example, some germs in the body help us break down the food we eat. If people did not have these germs, they would get sick.

Where are germs found?

Germs can be found in our hair, on our hands, on a pencil. There are germs almost everywhere.

How are germs passed from person to person?

Germs can be spread in different ways. One way is by touching things that have germs on them. Because germs cannot be seen, hands do not have to look dirty to have germs on them. This is why people should always wash their hands before eating.

People should be careful not to touch things likely to carry disease-causing germs, such as used drug needles, dead animals, animal droppings, things in trash cans, and other people's blood. Other objects, like used cups or forks, or a used tissue, might also have germs on them that could spread an illness.

Some germs, like cold germs, are spread through the air when people cough or sneeze. These germs live in the saliva and mucus of people's mouths and noses. When people cough or sneeze, small drops of the saliva and mucus go into the air and can spread to other people.

Some germs live in blood and are spread only through blood. Germs that are only spread this way are harder to pass from one person to another. These germs are not spread by cups or forks.

How can people prevent germs from being passed from person to person?

- Wash hands before meals, after playing outside, after touching something that might have germs.

- Do not touch things that are likely to have disease-causing germs on them, such as used drug needles, dead animals, animal droppings, things in trash cans, or other people's blood.

- Cover your mouth when coughing or sneezing, and then wash hands afterwards.

Unit 2, *continued*

Additional Information for Teachers

Disease-causing organisms ("pathogens") are classified into different types, including bacteria, viruses, fungi and parasites. Each of these different kinds of organisms has its own characteristics, and each can affect the body in different ways.

Treatment for different diseases depends to a large extent on the type of organism causing the illness. For example, bacteria-caused diseases can usually be treated with antibiotics. However, there are few effective treatments for viral diseases. In many cases, people with viral illnesses such as colds or the flu simply have to wait for the disease to run its course before the body is healthy again. For more serious viral diseases, such as HIV, there is no cure and only limited treatment is available.

Discussing Serious Illness with Young Children

TWO POINTS ARE HELPFUL to keep in mind in discussing serious illness with children. First, many children do or will have experience with serious illness (in a family member, friend or classmate), and they deserve clear and accurate information about this phenomenon. Second, because children tend to overgeneralize information, a discussion of serious illness is likely to raise anxieties about their own experiences with not-so-serious illnesses unless they can make a clear differentiation between the two.

Many of the same principles that are important in talking to children about death (see p. 193) also apply in discussing serious illness. Television and children's stories that make reference to illnesses may not make clear distinctions about what makes a serious illness different from a mild one. Children are understandably confused by the information they have gathered. Giving children a way to appreciate the distinctions between serious and not-so-serious illnesses can help prepare them for future experiences where it may be important for them to understand the difference.

We may not be able to answer all of children's questions about serious illnesses, but our willingness to respond shows them that we take their concerns seriously and reassures them that their questions are reasonable. Reassurance is an important theme. Children need to understand that most of the illnesses people have are not serious, and, in particular, most of the illnesses that affect children are not serious.

They need to know that parents or guardians know what signs to look for when they become sick, and will take them to a doctor if the illness needs treatment. And, while there are many things doctors do not know about specific illnesses (doctors do not know how to cure sickle cell disease or diabetes, for example), they do know how to tell

How AIDS Works: Grades K–3

Unit 2, *continued*

whether a person who is sick has a serious condition.

Children also need to understand that many visits to hospitals, outpatient surgery centers, or urgent care services are not the result of serious illnesses. Children may fear that individuals who go to such places have fatal conditions. Let them know that some not-so-serious conditions might require such a visit (having tonsils out, getting stitches after an injury, getting medicine for an illness when the regular doctor's office is closed), and that there are healthy reasons a person might go to a hospital (delivering a baby, having a checkup after recovering from a serious illness).

The story in the Evaluation for this unit ("Elizabeth and Mrs. Shaw") highlights some common misconceptions children may have about illnesses and provides opportunities to discuss the important concepts of differentiation (different causes, different symptoms, different treatments). Elizabeth's neighbor and friend, Mrs. Shaw, has cancer and is very sick. Elizabeth herself has strep throat and is taking medicine for it. She wonders why her medicine can't make Mrs. Shaw better, too.

Elizabeth is helped to understand the differences between her illness and its treatment and Mrs. Shaw's. In general, young children need a similar kind of assistance to reassure them that not every illness that affects them or people they care about is serious, and that most illnesses have straightforward and reliable treatments that help people recover fully.

Unit 3
Portals of Entry for Germs

OFTEN, STUDENTS BECOME ANXIOUS after lessons about germs and disease. The idea that invisible organisms are all over everything they see and touch may lead them to worry unnecessarily about the dangers of germs.

For this reason, it is important to explain and demonstrate that the body has many ways to protect itself from germs. Germs can only cause disease if they are able to get inside the body in some manner, and there are limited ways this can happen. The germs have to find an opening before they can enter the body.

The most common openings, or portals of entry, for germs are in the head: mouth, nose and eyes. Each opening has structures that help protect it from dirt, dust and germs.

Eyes

The eyes are protected by the eye sockets, which are inset, and the eyebrows, which help keep water, dirt and dust from getting in. Eyelids keep dirt and dust out of the eye when closed, and help wipe the surface of the eye clean every time a person blinks. Tears help wash away dirt, dust and germs.

Nose

The nose is lined with tiny hairs. When people breathe they produce a fine vapor. This environment stops most dirt, dust and pollen from getting inside the body through the nose. Mucus helps wash these materials away if they do get inside the nose.

Mouth

Saliva in the mouth actually has some germ-killing properties. Saliva can also help wash away dirt and dust. Coughing and sneezing carry away dirt, dust, pollen and germs, and the mucus produced during coughs or sneezes helps in this process.

Ears

Ears are a special case. Although it might look like there is an opening into the body through the ears, there is actually a thin piece of skin, the ear drum, at the end of the ear canal. The ear drum protects the inside of the body. It also makes it possible for a person to go swimming without getting water inside his or her head. The water can only go as far as the ear drum, and eventually comes back out. Ears also have tiny hairs and ear wax that help keep ear canals free of dirt and dust. The ear drum itself stays healthier in such an environment.

It is important not to put cotton swabs or other small items in the ears. Ears stay healthier when ear wax inside the ear canal is not disturbed. The tiny hairs in the ear actually move the wax to the outside of the canal, where it can easily be cleaned away. Use of cotton swabs inside the canal can compact the wax and lead to infection, perforation of the ear drum or other problems.

Most ear infections, however, are the result of germs entering through the mouth or nose and producing the symptom of swelling and inflammation in the middle ear.

Breaks in the Skin

Germs can also enter the body through irritations or breaks in the skin. This is why it is important to keep wounds clean and cover them if they will be exposed to dirt or other sources of germs.

Genital Openings

Some students may mention portals of entry associated with sexuality and elimination. While it is not necessary to bring these topics up in this unit, it will not hurt students to discuss them in the same direct, forthright manner that eyes and ears are being discussed. You will want to think about how to respond if a student asks about these openings in the discussion. Address student comments on this subject based on your school or district's guidelines concerning discussions of sexuality and body function.

Germs can enter the body through the vagina or the urethra (urinary opening) in women, through the urethra in the penis in men, and through the anus. Like the eyes, mouth, nose and ears, these openings have some built-in protections from germs. The penis has skin that closes around the opening and keeps out dirt and germs. The vagina and urethra in women also have folds of skin that protect the openings. The vagina has a moist substance similar to saliva that helps kill germs and keep the body clean. The anus has folds of skin that close up tight to keep out germs.

The Immune System

None of these systems for protecting portals from germs is foolproof. If germs do get past these barriers and inside the body, the immune system goes to work to keep the germs from causing damage and to clean them out of the body.

Unit 3, *continued*

Understanding the Immune System

YOUNG CHILDREN DO NOT need sophisticated knowledge about the immune system. However, children as young as age 5 have been able to understand in a general way that internal processes—helper cells in the blood—are at work to keep their bodies healthy, even though these cannot be seen, felt or heard.

An extremely simplified explanation of how the body protects itself from disease is presented in Unit 3. It is not necessary for you to have a scientific background or a more developed understanding of the immune system's processes. For purposes of this curriculum it will not be necessary to be familiar with anything more than a few general concepts.

Immune Responses

The body has 2 types of immune responses. *General responses* react to any pathogen detected. The general immune responses "go after everything"—all kinds of pathogens, microorganisms or particles that represent a threat to the body's health. *Specific responses* are linked to specific pathogens only. They are effective with those pathogens (a specific flu virus, for example), but have no effect on other pathogens.

General Responses

To fight pathogens quickly once they get inside the body, the immune system uses general response mechanisms. These mechanisms are always in place and on alert, so they can respond immediately to any pathogen.

- **Chemical defenses.** Pathogens that get inside the body are attacked by chemicals produced by a variety of body cells. For example, cells infected by viruses produce interferon, a family of proteins that protect other cells from the virus.

- **White blood cells.** There are a number of different types of white blood cells. Depending on the type and form, white blood cells might play a role in either general or specific immune responses.

  Phagocytes (FAG-o-sites) are white blood cells that respond to and neutralize a wide range of pathogens or particles in blood or tissue. They absorb and then ingest these microorganisms. In fact, the name of one type of phagocyte, "macrophage," comes from the Greek and means "big eater." They can migrate through blood vessel walls to fight infection.

  Phagocytes are one of the first lines of defense against infection, a sort of "sentry" of the immune system. In this role, they are part of the body's general immune response.

- **The inflammatory response.** To fight pathogens that get inside, the body concentrates phagocytes, other white blood cells and chemical defenses in an area of infection.

How AIDS Works: Grades K–3

Unit 3, continued

Specific Responses

In addition to the general responses to infection, special white blood cells can recognize and deactivate specific pathogens that enter the body, and "remember" them later to prevent future infection by the same pathogens. This is called the specific immune response.

Specific immune responses are extraordinary in their adaptability and effectiveness. They can identify and respond to *any* pathogen that enters the body, no matter how rare or unusual. Scientists have even manufactured entirely new particles for research purposes—structures that have never existed before—and immune system cells have been able to develop antibodies specifically linked to those particles.

The drawback to this very sophisticated system is that in each new case of infection, it takes some time for the body to produce enough of the necessary specialized cells to have an effect. This may be a period of a few hours to a couple of days. During this time, the general immune responses are particularly important in limiting or fighting infection.

The specific immune response involves different white blood cells. Each has a particular role in the immune response once a pathogen enters the body.

- **Phagocytes.** In their role as general immune system "sentries," phagocytes sometimes find a pathogen is too numerous or too strong to handle on their own. At that point, they signal other white blood cells, called *lymphocytes,* for help.

- **Lymphocytes.** Different lymphocytes have different functions during the immune response. Some (*helper T-cells*) identify pathogens. Others (*B-cells*) produce antibodies that weaken the pathogens so other white blood cells can kill them.

   The antibodies "mark" the pathogens with proteins that induce phagocytes to absorb them. These phagocytes are responding to specific pathogens—they have shifted roles and become mechanisms of the specific immune response.

   Other lymphocytes (*killer T-cells*) deal with viruses that have invaded and taken over cells in the body. Still others (*supressor T-cells*) turn off the immune response once the pathogen is defeated.

   Finally, some lymphocytes (*memory T-cells, memory B-cells*) remember the pathogen's form and "signature" so that if that specific pathogen returns the body can fight it more quickly and easily.

Unit 4
3 Points About AIDS

MANY TEACHERS WORRY THAT they do not know enough about AIDS to offer effective classroom instruction. While there is certainly an extraordinary amount of factual knowledge available about AIDS, what you need to know is practical and manageable. There are three basic ideas to communicate to students in this section of the curriculum.

1. AIDS is important because it is a serious disease that has affected many people's lives.

AIDS is considered a serious disease because its effects on the body can be profound, treatment options have limited impact on the course of the disease, and there is no cure. Over time, most people with HIV become progressively more ill, and many people have died of the disease.

Students themselves may know people who have HIV infection or who are caring for someone with AIDS.

2. The AIDS germ is different from other kinds of germs students may be familiar with.

You will want your students to understand that the way the AIDS germ passes from one person to another is very different from the way a cold or flu germ does. Cold and flu germs can be found almost "everywhere." The AIDS germ is found in only a few places—in blood and other special fluids inside the body. Cold and flu germs travel easily through the air, can be transmitted through coughs or sneezes, and can be picked up on hands by touching something that has the germs on it. The AIDS germ is only passed from person to person through activities where "inside-the-body" fluids are passed.

3. While some children do have AIDS, it is not a common disease among children.

Many children report concerns that they have AIDS, or might get it in the future. This curriculum stresses that each disease has unique qualities. For your students, the most important unique quality of AIDS is that the AIDS germ is different from other germs. When children understand the ways in which each illness is different, it will be easier for them to understand that while many people get colds, chicken pox and the flu, AIDS is a hard illness to get. In this unit, they will build the knowledge necessary to understand that most students their age do not do the kinds of things that pass the AIDS germ from person to person.

Guiding the Discussion

For the rest of the discussion, rely on your already-existing foundation of knowledge about AIDS. (See Background Information About HIV, p. 167.) Students may volunteer facts, guesses, rumors or blatant misconceptions. To the best of your

How AIDS Works: Grades K–3

Unit 4, *continued*

ability, confirm correct information and correct misinformation. (You will address transmission in greater detail in Activity 3 of this unit.) If students make statements you are not sure about, it is fine to acknowledge this. Set these questions aside for further research, and come back to the class with answers at a later time. An AIDS information line (either the National AIDS Information Hotline at 1-800-342-AIDS, or a local service) is an excellent resource for information.

The real skill in presenting this unit lies in your ability to weave these 3 important themes throughout the material. Students who are able to understand these points will be far better served than those taught by a teacher who is extremely knowledgeable about AIDS facts, but does not know how to present the facts in a way that emphasizes the larger and more important concepts.

Remember to keep discussions of AIDS simple. With children this age, it is not really necessary to clarify the distinctions between AIDS and asymptomatic HIV infection. Especially with younger elementary-age children, it is often preferable to let some of the finer points of scientific accuracy go, in order to present the material in a clear and easy-to-understand fashion.

Another example is the statement in this curriculum that "Mothers do *not* pass the AIDS germ to their children after they are born." There have been a few cases of HIV transmission to newborns through breast milk. For this reason, HIV-positive women in developed countries are advised to use formula for infant feeding. Technically, then, some women *have* passed HIV to offspring after birth. However, it is most important to emphasize that parents with HIV can care for and raise their children without putting them at risk for the illness.

Talking About AIDS Transmission with Early Elementary Students

WHEN DISCUSSING AIDS with young children, adults naturally look for simple, straightforward language that will inform without confusing. However, if we choose terms and language that "protect" children, we may leave out important pieces of information.

A good example would be the use of the term "sleeping together" to describe sexual intercourse. While young children may be familiar with this term, most are probably not clear on the actual meaning. They may worry that sharing a bed with a sibling puts them at risk for AIDS.

It is important to think ahead of time of terms and language you can use to discuss AIDS that will be comfortable for you to use, clear and thorough for the children, and meet the guidelines and standards of your school or district. In

Unit 4, *continued*

this curriculum, the term "close sexual contact" is used in discussions of HIV transmission, and is clarified by explaining that this does *not* mean hugging and kissing.

When frank discussions like this are taking place, some students may ask questions that increase the explicitness of the material (e.g., "Do people get AIDS when the condom falls off?"). The Guidelines for Discussing Sensitive Topics (p. 186) offer some help in this regard. Decide ahead of time on the terms you prefer to use for discussions, and think about how you will handle sensitive questions if they come up.

Children's Understanding of Drugs and AIDS

MOST SCHOOL CHILDREN TODAY have had drug abuse prevention education and smoking prevention education. Even children in early elementary grades are familiar with the ideas that drugs are dangerous, that they make people sick, and that children and adults should avoid using drugs.

Lessons about AIDS may draw on what students already know about drug use. However, because young children tend to overgeneralize in evaluating new information, particular misunderstandings may arise during lessons about AIDS. The guidelines given here can help you avoid the most common misconceptions that arise when discussing drug use and AIDS with young children.

Help children understand that, while drugs make people sick in many ways, they do not *cause* AIDS. Children may already know that using drugs can make people sick. They also know that drug use is associated in some way with AIDS. A common misunderstanding is that the drugs actually *cause* AIDS. This can lead to fears that family members or friends who use drugs (cigarettes, alcohol, marijuana) might develop AIDS.

When children understand the concepts in this curriculum, they will be better prepared to understand the connection between drug use and AIDS: People who use needles (syringes) to take drugs, and who share these needles with others, may be exposed to small amounts of other people's blood. The AIDS germ lives in blood. Therefore, it is the AIDS germ, in the blood, in the needle, that causes AIDS—not the drugs themselves.

Reassure children that any shots they receive for medical purposes are safe. Children who know that the AIDS germ may be found in syringes may not understand that the syringes used at medical clinics and doctor's offices are sterile. In any discussion of AIDS transmission through injection drug needles, it is important to reassure children that needles used in medical settings are only used on one person, then are thrown

How AIDS Works: Grades K–3

Unit 4, *continued*

away. Children cannot get AIDS from getting a shot at a doctor's office.

Check children's understanding. Look for signs of concrete thinking. Children often hear phrases that have clear meaning for adults and apply very concrete interpretations to these. A good example is the term "dirty needles." To AIDS educators, drug treatment providers and drug users, this term refers to injection drug needles that have been shared. To children, it may suggest a syringe, or even a sewing needle, that is literally dirty—that is, a needle with dirt on it.

An unfortunate trend in recent years is the discarding of used syringes in sandlots or elsewhere in playgrounds. It is important that children be aware that they might find syringes in these places and know to find an adult to help out if they do. However, when young children are warned to watch for "dirty" needles on the playground, it may lead to confusion. If dirt in a needle can cause AIDS, can dirt on someone's hands cause AIDS?

It is important to check children's comprehension thoroughly, and to ask questions that encourage them to explain in some detail how they are applying their new knowledge. Responses that simply parrot back phrases they have heard ("AIDS is caused by dirty needles") do not give you an opportunity to evaluate whether a child actually understands the underlying concepts.

Offer reassurance and resources to children if they raise concerns about family members' use of cigarettes, alcohol or other drugs. Lessons that address drug use may raise specific concerns for some children. Be prepared to offer individual attention to children who have special concerns about drug use in their families and make referrals for further assessment if substance abuse problems in the home seem possible.

Note: The assumption of this curriculum is that students will have already had some background in drug prevention and that these lessons on illnesses and AIDS will not be their first introduction to the topic. See Addressing Drug Use and AIDS (p. 198) for suggestions for reviewing issues concerning drug use if students have not already covered this material. However, this information is provided with a *strong* recommendation that a separate curriculum address this important topic in more depth.

Unit 5
Preventing AIDS: Important Concepts for Children

WHEN OFFERING HIV EDUCATION to elementary-age students, many questions may arise. How much should be said? What are the right points to emphasize and how much repetition is appropriate? Is it really necessary to discuss sexuality and injection drug use? Must these be mentioned more than once?

Remember that many children, even at the lowest grade levels, have already heard about sex and drugs as causes of AIDS. And, in many cases, their understanding is limited or inaccurate. Therefore, it is important to present and clarify these modes of transmission in classroom education about AIDS. Three steps will help in this effort.

Be Clear About Concepts

First, be clear about the important concepts and facts for young children to know about AIDS. This curriculum emphasizes the following:

- The AIDS germ is a special kind of germ. It is an "inside" germ, and is not easily passed from one person to another.

- The AIDS germ can only be passed from one person to another through a few activities: blood-to-blood contact, mother-to-baby during pregnancy and delivery, close sexual contact, or sharing needles for taking drugs. Most students in elementary school do not do these things. This is why they do not need to worry about having or getting AIDS.

- The AIDS germ damages the immune system. This makes it hard for the body to fight off other diseases.

- There are simple steps people can take to protect themselves from AIDS.

- There are just a few things that are important for children to know to protect themselves from AIDS. These include avoiding all kinds of blood-to-blood contact, not sharing needles for drug use or other reasons, and not having sex. Grown-ups know how to protect themselves from the AIDS germ when they have sex.

Be Familiar with Common Misconceptions

Second, be familiar with the common misconceptions children may develop about AIDS. In particular, be aware of the following possible misunderstandings:

- Drugs themselves causing AIDS; for example, believing that alcohol or cigarettes might give someone AIDS.

- Casual contact being considered a risk because children believe that some kinds of casual contact (hugging, kissing, sharing a bed) are a form of having sex.

- The AIDS germ behaving like other

How AIDS Works: Grades K–3

Unit 5, *continued*

familiar germs (colds and flus), and being easy to transmit.
- Minor illnesses possibly being serious, or even life-threatening, as AIDS is.

Actively Engage Students

Third, develop teaching strategies that actively engage children in the learning, allow you to measure their comprehension and offer you the opportunity to clarify information and correct misconceptions. Two helpful approaches in this regard include:

- Use thoughtfully worded questions that encourage children to express their understanding more fully. For example, if a child says, "Drugs cause AIDS," ask an open-ended question: "And how is it that drugs can cause AIDS?" The child's response will let you know whether this is a statement of true comprehension (infected blood in shared needles can pass the virus from one person to another), or the parroting of a "fact" learned from television or other sources.

- Use clarifying statements that anticipate children's misconceptions. For example, if a child says, "People can get AIDS from sex," you might respond, "Yes. This is one way people can get the AIDS germ. And of course, when we talk about sex, we are talking about close sexual contact. This does not include kissing, hugging or holding hands. We do not need to worry about catching AIDS from these things."

Many children will come to the first lesson with misconceptions about communicable diseases in general and AIDS specifically. It helps to anticipate this. No matter how well the lessons are taught, further misconceptions are bound to arise. It is important to view children's expression of these misconceptions as signs of success. It shows that the children are actively engaged in the learning process and that they feel safe enough to reveal the limits of their knowledge. It also provides a forum for correcting misunderstandings and building skills in differentiation.

The most effective teaching environment will examine closely the true extent of children's comprehension and use every opportunity to advance their knowledge and understanding.

Unit 6
Guest Speakers, Videos and Stories

IN UNIT 6, YOU MAY CHOOSE to invite a guest speaker, show a video or read a story to the class. There are many books and videos currently available for elementary school age children on the topic of AIDS. The Selected Resources (p. 200) lists some of the most useful ones. Many more resources will become available over the next several years. For current resources, check with the librarian of your school or public library.

Videos and Stories

Here are some general guidelines for selecting an appropriate video or story for your class:

- **Language.** Is the language appropriate to students' developmental level? Language should be clear, and information should be stated succinctly and in simple terms. Avoid films or stories that use medical jargon or terms that young children do not, *and need not*, understand.

    Evaluate the way language is used to deliver information. For example, several films for young children use songs, poems or rap to convey important information. Unfortunately, clarity is too often sacrificed for the sake of selecting a rhyming word or a phrase containing the right number of syllables. This is not a wise approach if the cost is lack of accuracy.

- **Ways HIV is transmitted.** Are all 4 of the major ways HIV is spread—close sexual contact, blood-to-blood contact, sharing needles for injection drug use or other purposes, mother to infant during pregnancy and delivery—presented? If not, you may still wish to use the story or video, but be sure to supplement the information as necessary.

- **Something new or different.** Does the film or story do something that you cannot do yourself in class? For example, a video that shows children who have HIV allows the class to see that children with HIV can look and act like other children and, perhaps most important, have feelings just like other children. Such materials may help enhance children's empathy and dispel myths.

- **Reinforce learning.** Does the information reinforce what you have already taught? Is the information provided in a way that promotes further understanding, rather than just attempting to teach more facts?

- **Cultural or gender bias.** Is the material free of any cultural or gender bias? Although it is not necessary for the film or story to depict individuals of every culture or background, it is preferable that some diversity be present. Cartoons with race-neutral characters represent one solution.

How AIDS Works: Grades K–3

Unit 6, *continued*

- **Does the presentation work?** Is the story engaging? Is the production quality high? Will this material sustain children's attention? A film in excess of 15–20 minutes may need to be shown over more than one session.

- **Do you like the film or the story?** Chances are that if you do not like the material, your class won't either.

Guest Speakers

You could also invite a guest speaker to address the class: an adult with HIV, an older student with HIV (middle or high school age), someone who has a family member affected, a nurse or doctor who works with people with HIV, or an educator or counselor specializing in HIV. The most important criteria for selecting a speaker to talk with young children include the following:

- **Ability to communicate clearly and appropriately.** Can this person speak at a level young children can understand? Will he or she address topics appropriate to their interest? Can the speaker talk about broader concepts as well as technical facts?

- **Engaging personal style.** Does this speaker have an engaging manner? Is this someone you like to listen to? If you do not find the speaker interesting, chances are your students will feel similarly.

- **Availability to hear about what the students already know.** Can the speaker spend time talking with you to find out what has been covered in the curriculum? This accomplishes 2 things: it orients the speaker to the level of learning students have achieved, and it familiarizes the speaker with language and terms used in the class. The speaker can then use language familiar to the students in the presentation and reach them more effectively.

- **Sufficient detachment from the subject.** Some speakers bring a personal agenda to their presentations—they want people to understand, agree with or commit to something. It is important for a speaker to understand something about the ways young children think and communicate about the world, and to accept both the richness and the limitations of that communication.

    For example, a speaker who can help children discuss their feelings and attitudes openly might effectively help them build empathy towards people with HIV. But a speaker who insists from the outset that students accept people with HIV completely and without prejudice may not be as persuasive or helpful.

There are many ways a speaker could proceed. A suggested set-up is to introduce the speaker, including why he or she was invited to speak to the class; have the speaker talk for 5 minutes or less; and then invite students to ask questions, allowing this question-and-answer session to make up the bulk of the presentation.

Review Guide

REVIEWING CONCEPTS from previous units briefly at the beginning of each new unit is an important component of this curriculum. Review segments are built into each unit. Unit 2 reviews the important concepts delivered in Unit 1; Unit 3 reviews the important concepts delivered in Units 1 and 2; and so on.

These review segments are intentionally repetitive. Children are quite capable of learning the concepts included in this curriculum. However, this kind of learning will be new for many students and will require frequent repetition and reinforcement to be solidly acquired.

It takes children longer to comprehend broad concepts than to learn simple facts. Therefore, it is important to give students ample opportunity to practice and apply this new kind of knowledge. The review segments allow them to do this.

At the start of each unit, children should hear that different illnesses have different ways someone gets them; that different illnesses make people sick in different ways; and that there are different things people can do to get better from different illnesses. Throughout the lessons, challenge students to apply any new information to their already acquired knowledge of these concepts.

For example, in the review in Unit 2, you could ask the class, "What is something different between stomach flu and an asthma attack?" Students who understand the concepts presented in Unit 1 may say that you can catch a flu from someone, but you cannot catch asthma. When reviewing these same concepts in Unit 3, you might ask the question in a more sophisticated manner: "Can someone name 2 different illnesses and then tell me something that's different between them?" The same concepts are being reviewed, but students are being asked to apply their knowledge in a more complex way.

As new information is introduced, take every opportunity to reemphasize and repeat the general concepts of each unit. For example, in Unit 4, when introducing the fact that HIV lives in blood and certain body fluids and can be spread through the transfer of these fluids, you can state, "This is one way the AIDS germ is 'different' from other germs. Cold germs live in saliva and are spread when saliva is passed from a person with a cold to someone else. The AIDS germ lives in blood and certain body fluids. It can spread only when these fluids are passed from a person with the AIDS germ to someone else."

Questions are provided as a guide to reviewing the main points presented in each unit.

How AIDS Works: Grades K–3

Unit 1: Different Illnesses

1. We've talked about many ways that illnesses are different. What are some of the important differences we have talked about?

   Different causes (There are different ways someone gets them.)

   Different symptoms (Each illness makes people sick in different ways.)

   Different treatments (There are different things people can do to get better from different illnesses.)

2. When would a person need to be careful not to catch an illness from someone who is sick?

   Some illnesses one person can catch from another; some illnesses one person cannot catch from another. A person would need to be careful not to catch an illness from someone if it is the kind of illness that can be passed from one person to another.

Unit 2: Different Ways to Be Sick

1. In what kinds of places do germs live?

   Some germs can live almost anywhere; other germs can only live in a few places.

2. What kinds of things can people do to keep from getting illnesses that are easy-to-pass, such as colds?

   Avoid close, casual contact—sharing eating utensils, touching hands after someone has coughed into his or her hand, someone coughing nearby.

3. Can every illness pass from one person to another this easily?

   No, some diseases are easy to pass, but others are hard to pass.

4. Remember when we heard the story about Elizabeth and Mrs. Shaw? Elizabeth had strep throat. She found out that her illness was not serious. How did she know this?

   It wasn't going to last very long. Medicines would help cure it. She did not feel very bad. She would get better soon. She was only missing a few days of school.

   Elizabeth's neighbor, Mrs. Shaw, had cancer. How did Elizabeth know that Mrs. Shaw's illness was serious?

   Mrs. Shaw had been sick a long time. The medicines were not making her better right away. The doctor did not know how long she would be sick. She had been unable to work for a long time.

Unit 3: How the Body Stays Well

1. A germ has to do something to make a person sick. What does a germ need to do?

   A germ must get inside the body to make a person sick.

2. What are some ways germs can get inside a person's body?

   Common portals of entry include the mouth, nose, eyes, cuts in the skin.

3. Our bodies have many ways to protect themselves from germs. What are some of these ways?

   Skin; hairs in the nose; the ear drum; coughing and sneezing; saliva washing out germs, dirt and dust; eyelids and eyebrows; ear wax; helper cells in the blood. Help students differentiate between "outside" and "inside" ways the body protects itself.

Unit 4: What About AIDS?

1. What are some of the important things we learned about AIDS?

   AIDS is an "inside germ;" it is not easily passed from one person to another. It can only be passed from one person to another through a few activities, and these are not common among elementary-age children. The AIDS germ damages the immune system, interfering with the body's ability to fight off other diseases.

2. What are the ways the AIDS germ can be passed from person to person?

   Blood-to-blood contact

   Mother-to-baby transmission

   Close sexual contact

   Sharing needles for taking drugs

Unit 5: Preventing AIDS

1. What are the most important things for children to know about AIDS?

   Children this age don't usually get AIDS. Children don't usually do the kinds of things that can pass the AIDS germ. Don't touch blood. Don't touch used syringes. It's OK to have questions about AIDS. There are grown-ups who can help answer questions about AIDS.

2. What kinds of things can people do to keep from getting AIDS?

   Keep the AIDS germ from getting inside their body. Don't touch blood. Don't touch used syringes. Don't share needles for taking drugs. Don't have sex. Grown-ups have ways to have sex that can protect them from the AIDS germ.

Unit 6: Helping Out

In Unit 6, review all concepts from previous units with students.

How AIDS Works: Grades K–3

Information for Parents

TO HELP YOU WELCOME parent input and involve parents directly in their children's classroom experiences, this section includes guidelines for notifying parents about the AIDS curriculum, along with a sample notification letter that can be adapted to meet the needs and requirements of your particular school or district. There is also a handout that can be sent home to parents, either with the notificaton letter, or at whatever point in the lessons you feel is most appropriate. **About AIDS and HIV: Background Information for Parents** explains what HIV/AIDS is, how it's transmitted and how people can protect themselves. This handout includes information for adults, as well as language and suggestions to help parents respond to their children's questions. It can be adapted to meet the needs and requirements of your particular school or district.

Parent Notification

Many states have parental notification requirements regarding sexuality education. The following list of guidelines may be helpful in preparing your parental notification letter. The sample letter provided is meant as an example only; adapt it to meet the needs and requirements of your district.

Letters should be timely, specific, positive and concise:

- **Timely.** Be sure to allow parents adequate time to review materials, meet with the teacher or attend any parent preview meetings.
  - Announcement of any meetings should reach parents at least 2 weeks before the meeting.
  - Notification that the child is in the class should occur at least 3 weeks before the course begins.
  - If written parental permission is required, ample time to collect the permission slips should be allowed.
- **Specific.** Parents need to know what topic areas will be covered and what types of approaches will be used in order to make an informed decision about their child's participation in the course. If possible, attach a complete course outline to the letter.
- **Positive.** For many parents, the parent notification letter will be their only acquaintance with the course or the teacher. It is your opportunity to communicate your respect for the values of the home and family, as well as your commitment to the course.
- **Concise.** Give parents the information that they need in a clear, concise, readable style.

SAMPLE LETTER

Sample Parent Notification Letter

Dear Parents,

We are pleased to inform you that your child will be offered a curriculum on AIDS education in his/her class this semester. The curriculum will begin on _____ . Each unit includes several different
              [date]
activities, presented over a period of several days.

The Curriculum

The name of the curriculum is "How AIDS Works." It was written by a pediatrician and a family counselor, and tested in classrooms before it was published.

Many AIDS curricula simply teach facts about AIDS. This curriculum is different because it emphasizes *concepts*. Concepts are broad ideas that apply to many different circumstances. They provide a framework students can use to judge further information.

For example, after completing these lessons, a student who hears incorrect ideas about AIDS from a playmate will have skills to evaluate the information, and will probably know that it is wrong. What your child will learn will provide a good foundation for additional learning and thoughtful evaluation of this important issue in future years.

Topics Covered

The lessons will cover a variety of topics, presented in an age-appropriate manner, including:

- ways illnesses are different
- some of the ways illnesses can be passed from one person to another
- how the AIDS germ is different from other germs children often hear about
- the ways the AIDS germ can be passed
- how people can protect themselves from AIDS

Teaching techniques will include lectures, storytelling, demonstrations, and completing activity sheets or drawings.

(continued)

How AIDS Works: Grades K–3

SAMPLE LETTER

continued

Family Homework

At the end of each unit, students will bring home a letter. The letter will describe what students are learning and list the concepts they have been taught. It will also suggest some questions you can ask your child about the lessons.

We hope you will complete these family activities with your child. Students will not be asked to report back to the class, but talking with you will help reinforce what your child has learned. The family activities also give you a time to discuss your own family's values about the topics.

Preview Meetings

There will be a parent preview meeting before the curriculum begins. At this meeting, you will be able to meet the teacher, review the lessons and learn more about the content and goals of the class. The meeting will be held _____. We strongly encourage you to attend.
 [date, time, location]

If you are unable to attend the meeting but would like to review the class materials, please contact the school and we will arrange a preview time. I am available to answer any of your questions or concerns.

Permission to Participate

If you choose *not* to have your child participate in the AIDS curriculum, please sign the form below and return it to the school as soon as possible so we can arrange an alternate learning activity for your child. If we do not hear from you by _____, we will assume you approve
 [date class is starting]
of your child's participation in the course.

We hope to see you at the parent preview.

        Sincerely,

        _____
                [Principal or teacher]

Please excuse my child, _____ ,
                    [student name]
from the AIDS curriculum. I understand that he/she will participate in an appropriate alternate learning activity during these class times.

_____   _____
   [date]   [signature of Parent/Guardian]

FAMILY HANDOUT

About AIDS and HIV: Background Information for Parents

Dear Parents,

Your child is about to begin a series of classroom lessons about AIDS. Students are encouraged to discuss these lessons with their parents.

This handout gives basic information about HIV and AIDS. It is written for adults and covers more detail than your child's classes will. However, you may find this information helpful in answering any questions about AIDS your child might raise at home.

Suggestions for talking about the topics with children are included. The "Key points" for each section cover the content of the classroom lessons. These key points are useful to emphasize when talking with your child. Feel free to change how you phrase your answers to match your child's age, level of understanding and your own family's values.

What Is AIDS? What Is HIV?
Information for Adults

AIDS is a disease that breaks down the body's immune system. When this happens, the body cannot fight off certain kinds of illnesses. A person might get one or more unusual, life-threatening diseases.

HIV is the name of the virus that causes AIDS. It stands for "human immunodeficiency virus."

People may be infected with HIV for many years before they develop signs or symptoms of illness. You cannot tell just by looking at someone whether he or she has HIV or AIDS. An AIDS diagnosis is usually given at an advanced stage of HIV infection.

What to Say to Children

AIDS is a serious disease that some people get. It can make them very sick. Fortunately, it is also a very hard disease to get. You can't get it the easy way you get colds or flu. We're glad about that, because it means you and I can protect ourselves from AIDS. Children your age almost never get AIDS.

(continued)

How AIDS Works: Grades K–3

FAMILY HANDOUT

continued

Key points:

- Most children do not get AIDS.
- Many children worry that they might get AIDS. Reassure your child about these concerns.

How Do People Get HIV?
Information for Adults

HIV lives in certain body fluids, especially blood, semen and vaginal fluids. People become infected with HIV by taking the blood, semen or vaginal fluids of an infected person into their bodies. There are 4 ways this might happen:

1. **Sexual intercourse:** People may take in the semen, vaginal fluids or blood of a sexual partner during vaginal, oral and anal intercourse, and pass or receive HIV in this way. Use of condoms or latex barriers can reduce this risk, though some risk remains because of the chance that these barriers could tear, break or fall off.

2. **Sharing needles or syringes:** When injection drug users share needles, small amounts of blood may remain in the needle or syringe as it is passed from person to person. Sharing needles for other reasons, like tattooing, ear or body piercing, or injecting steroids or insulin, is also risky. Syringes used in medical settings, like doctor's offices, are disposable. Because they are used on only one person and then thrown away, getting shots in a medical setting does not pose a risk for HIV.

3. **From an infected woman to her fetus or newborn:** A pregnant woman with HIV can pass the virus on to her fetus or newborn. Medications during pregnancy can lower, but not eliminate, this risk.

4. **Through infected blood or other internal body fluids or tissues:** In the past, some people were infected with HIV through blood transfusions or blood products. Now, a special test is used to screen blood donations for HIV. The risk of HIV in a blood transfusion today is very small—about 1 in 100,000. There is no risk in *donating* blood.

    A few cases of HIV have also been traced to human organ transplants and donor inseminations. Again, organ and semen donors are now tested for HIV. Finally, some health care workers have become infected with HIV through work-related accidents where they were stuck with needles or exposed to blood from a patient with HIV. Established infection control guidelines can help prevent such accidents.

(continued)

People do *not* get HIV in casual, day-to-day contact with family, friends, acquaintances, workmates or the population at large.

What to Say to Children

Like many diseases, AIDS is caused by a germ. The AIDS germ can only live inside the body. It can live in blood. It cannot live on the skin.

Most people have gotten AIDS either by having sex (sexual intercourse) with someone who has the AIDS germ, or by using needles to take drugs and sharing the needles with someone who has the AIDS germ. "Sex" does not mean kissing, hugging or holding hands.

There are only a few ways the AIDS germ can get from the inside of one person's body to the inside of another person's body. People do not get the AIDS germ from everyday contact with their family and friends.

Key points:

- There are only a few ways the AIDS germ can be passed from one person to another. If people don't do these things, they can protect themselves from the AIDS germ and don't need to worry about getting AIDS.
- People do not get the AIDS germ through everyday contact with others. You cannot get AIDS from hugging, sharing food or playing with someone.

How Can People Protect Themselves from HIV?
Information for Adults

The ways to prevent HIV are clear and straightforward.

1. Abstinence—not having sex with anyone—is the surest way to prevent the sexual transmission of HIV. People can also be monogamous—have sex with only one lifetime partner, who has never had sex with anyone else or shared needles.

2. Adults who choose to have sex in other situations can reduce the risk of HIV by using condoms or latex barriers for all types of intercourse.

3. People should never share needles or other equipment for injection drug use, ear or body piercing, tattooing or any other purpose.

4. Pregnant women with HIV, or who are at risk for HIV, should see a knowledgeable health care provider.

(continued)

FAMILY HANDOUT
continued

5. Health care workers should follow universal precautions for avoiding the transmission of bloodborne diseases. Other people should avoid touching blood in first-aid situations.

What to Say to Children

Because the AIDS germ can live in blood, you should not touch someone else's blood if he or she is hurt. Do not touch a drug needle if you find one on the ground or anywhere else. Get a grown-up to help.

If people don't have sex with anyone and don't use needles to take drugs, they don't need to worry about getting AIDS.

We can all live well without using drugs. Most grown-ups *do* want to have sex sometimes. But grown-ups know ways to protect themselves from getting the AIDS germ when they have sex.

Key points:

- "Sex" is not the same thing as hugging, kissing or holding hands. You cannot get AIDS from these things.
- Sharing needles to inject drugs can cause AIDS. Blood left in a needle when a person shares needles to inject drugs can have the AIDS germ in it. Drugs can make people sick in many ways, but drugs themselves do not cause AIDS.
- If someone is hurt and bleeding, get a grown-up to help. It's best not to touch anyone else's blood. Do not touch used drug needles.

For more information about AIDS, call the National AIDS Hotline at 1-800-342-AIDS.

Background Information About HIV

READING THIS BACKGROUND information about HIV and AIDS will give you a general understanding of the disease and the epidemic. Having this foundation of knowledge will help you provide better classroom education about AIDS. Much of this information is more sophisticated than your classroom discussions will be, however, and these answers are not recommended for use with young students.

General Information

What is AIDS? What is HIV?

AIDS is a disease that breaks down a part of the body's immune system, leaving a person vulnerable to a variety of unusual, life-threatening illnesses. People with AIDS may also suffer from neurologic problems, including forgetfulness, difficulty walking and confusion.

HIV is the name of the virus that causes AIDS. "HIV" stands for "human immunodeficiency virus." People may be infected with HIV for many years before they develop signs or symptoms of illness.

What is the difference between HIV infection and AIDS?

Anyone infected with HIV has HIV infection. This might include people with no physical symptoms, people with mild physical symptoms or people with severe physical symptoms.

An AIDS diagnosis is given when an individual with HIV infection has developed signs or symptoms of severe immune system impairment. Usually this is at an advanced stage of HIV infection.

What happens to the immune system when someone has HIV?

When a foreign organism enters the body of a person with a healthy immune system, the immune system identifies the intruder, mobilizes defenses against it, and establishes an ongoing specific "watch" to protect against that intruder in the future.

When a person has HIV infection, any part of this sequence may be disrupted. The immune system may not be able to recognize that a foreign organism has entered the body. If it does, it may be unable to mobilize defenses against it. If the defenses are mobilized, they may not function properly. And, finally, the body may be unable to establish a watch system against the intruder in the future.

For example, *Pneumocystis carinii* pneumonia is a common and serious infection in persons with HIV. It is caused by an organism which is all around us. Most of us have been exposed to this organism several times in our lives. With a healthy immune system, the body identifies and overwhelms the organism, and the person never becomes ill with the infection. For a person with HIV, the body may identify the organism, but seems unable to mount an effective defense. The infection takes hold and the person becomes seriously ill.

How long can a person be infected with HIV before being diagnosed with AIDS?

The length of time from first infection to diagnosis with AIDS, sometimes called the "incubation period" for AIDS, varies. In rare cases, it may be as little as a few weeks or months. Other people have had HIV infection for 15 years or longer, and still do not have an AIDS diagnosis. The average length of the incubation period is about 10 years.

Transmission

How do people get HIV?

HIV lives in certain body fluids, especially blood, semen and vaginal fluids. People become infected with HIV by taking the blood, semen or vaginal fluids of an infected person into their body. There are 4 ways this might happen:

- **Unprotected sexual intercourse.** People may take in the blood, semen or vaginal fluids of a sexual partner during vaginal, oral or anal intercourse. "Unprotected" intercourse means no condom or latex barrier was used.

- **Sharing needles or other equipment in injection drug use.** Injection drug users frequently share needles. Small amounts of blood may remain in a needle or syringe as it is passed from person to person. Sharing needles for other purposes (tattooing, ear or body piercing, injecting steroids or insulin) is also risky.

- **From an infected woman to her fetus or newborn.** A pregnant woman with HIV has an approximately 25% chance of passing the virus to her fetus or newborn. Medications taken during pregnancy and at the time of delivery can help protect the fetus from infection, though some risk of transmission remains. There are a few cases where a woman with HIV has transmitted the virus to her baby through her breast milk.

- **Through infected blood or other internal body fluids or tissues.** In the early 1980s, a number of people were infected with HIV through blood transfusions, and people with hemophilia were infected through being treated with medicines manufactured from human blood. Today, medicines for hemophilia are manufactured so they cannot transmit HIV, and, since 1985, blood donated for transfusions has been tested for HIV.

A few cases of HIV transmission have been traced to human organ transplants—organs were transplanted from a person with HIV and the recipient later developed the disease. Screening procedures are now in place to prevent this.

Some health care workers have

become infected with HIV through being stuck with infected needles or exposed to the blood or internal fluids of persons with HIV. Established infection control guidelines can help prevent accidents such as these.

People do *not* get HIV from day-to-day, casual contact with family, friends, acquaintances, workmates or the population at large.

Which body fluids carry HIV?

HIV has been found in a number of different body fluids. These include:

- blood
- any body fluid containing visible blood
- semen and pre-ejaculate
- vaginal fluids (vaginal or cervical secretions)
- menstrual blood
- human breast milk

Internal fluids that surround joints, organs or membranes also carry HIV. Health care workers should take precautions around such fluids, but other people are unlikely to have contact with them.

HIV has also been detected in a few other body fluids, but the concentration of the virus is so small that these fluids are not a danger. We do not need to worry about tears, saliva, urine, feces, vomit, nasal secretions, sputum or sweat, unless visible blood is present.

Can people get HIV through oral sex?

Yes. There are several documented cases of HIV transmission through oral sex in the medical literature. Most have involved taking semen or pre-ejaculate into the mouth. However, some individuals with HIV have said their only risk factor was having oral sex performed on them by a person with HIV.

Vaginal fluids and menstrual blood carry HIV. Therefore, oral sex performed on a woman with HIV should be considered a risky activity.

While the overall risk of oral sex is much lower than unprotected anal or vaginal intercourse, oral sex involves a genuine risk for a very serious disease.

Can people get HIV from insect bites?

No. There has never been a documented case of HIV transmission associated with insect bites, although many researchers have looked carefully for such evidence. Epidemiologic studies (who gets HIV, how and where) throughout the world reinforce researchers' findings:

- Consistently, people who have HIV also have some other identifiable risk activity, such as unprotected sexual intercourse with an infected person, sharing of needles, or being born to a mother with HIV.

- The population of people bitten by insects includes large numbers of children ages 6 to 12. Children this age are rarely diagnosed with AIDS, and those who are have identifiable risks.

- Studies of thousands of people with AIDS and HIV have shown transmission within households only where identifiable risks have occurred—for example, when a man and woman have had unprotected sexual intercourse. Household members who might presumably be bitten by the same insects have not developed HIV.

Can people still get HIV from blood transfusions?

The risk of contracting HIV through a blood transfusion is extremely small. Most people at known risk for HIV voluntarily avoid donating blood, and all blood in the United States donated for medical purposes is tested for HIV. While it is possible a donor with HIV could give blood during the "window period," before antibodies show up on a test, estimates of the actual risk of a given unit of blood being infected with HIV range from 1 in 40,000 to about 1 in 100,000.

Blood can carry a number of different human viruses, including HIV, hepatitis-B, and other forms of hepatitis. Because of the potential for infections to be transmitted during blood transfusions, physicians today recommend transfusions only when absolutely necessary. For elective surgeries, people are often able to arrange to "donate" their own blood beforehand, to preclude any chance of new infections being introduced into the body.

Can people get HIV from kissing?

There has never been a documented case of HIV transmission through kissing.

Any risk with kissing is not due to the exchange of saliva. Quantities of HIV in saliva are too small to cause infection. However, if both people had open sores or lesions in the mouth, bleeding gums, or other oral injuries, it is possible for HIV to be transmitted through an exchange of blood. In very vigorous, deep kissing, blood could be drawn, and this also poses a theoretical risk.

Is it safe to go to the dentist or doctor?

Yes. Doctors and dentists today are aware of the importance of infection control in a medical office. The only documented cases of HIV transmission within a medical setting all happened at the office of one dentist. No one is sure why this happened, because the dentist himself has since died. However, it is clear that something very unusual and improper took place in these cases.

Who Is at Risk?

Who can become infected with HIV?

Anyone can become infected with HIV if he or she has unprotected sexual intercourse or shares needles with someone else who is infected.

Are heterosexuals at risk for HIV?

Yes. While most cases of AIDS in the United States today are diagnosed among gay men or injection drug users, the percentage of people whose only risk factor is heterosexual contact has grown. In 1984, fewer than 1% of all AIDS cases were heterosexual transmission cases—about 50 people. By the end of 1994, 7% of all adolescent and adult AIDS cases were heterosexual transmission cases—about 32,000 people.

In many other countries, HIV is transmitted primarily through heterosexual contact.

The relative risk for heterosexuals in most parts of the United States today is small. Those at highest risk are people with multiple sex partners in areas where HIV is already widespread. Heterosexuals, like other people, can keep their risk lower by following safer sex guidelines and not sharing needles.

Are lesbians at risk for HIV?

Yes. Lesbians can contract HIV the same way anyone else can: by taking the blood, semen or vaginal fluids of an infected person into their bodies. Some lesbians have had past sexual relationships with men. Some have current sexual relationships with men. Others have used donor insemination to conceive a pregnancy. If male partners in any of these instances had HIV, there would be an HIV risk for the woman. There are also lesbians who have shared needles in injection drug use or other activities.

The sexual partners of a lesbian woman with HIV are at risk.

Are teenagers at risk for HIV?

Yes. Teenagers often experiment with drugs and sexual behavior. Some are sexually active with a number of different partners. Condom use, while increasing among teens, is still not widespread.

Because a person may have HIV for many years before being diagnosed with AIDS, the number of teenagers with AIDS is much lower than the number of teenagers with HIV.

At the end of 1994, over 16,000 teenagers and young adults (under age 25) had been diagnosed with AIDS. Most of the young adults were probably infected during their teens.

These figures make it clear that HIV prevention education for teenagers is especially important.

Avoiding HIV Infection

How can people protect themselves from HIV?

- Do not have unprotected intercourse (vaginal, oral or anal) with anyone unless you are *certain* the person does not have HIV. If there is any doubt, use condoms or latex barriers, or avoid intercourse.

- Never share needles or other equipment for injection drug use, injecting steroids or vitamins, ear or body piercing, tattooing or any other purpose.

- Health care workers should follow universal precautions for avoiding the transmission of bloodborne diseases.

What is safer sex?

Safer sex involves sexual activities that carry little or no risk of passing blood, semen or vaginal fluids between partners.

Some safer sex activities include:

- Masturbation, alone or with a partner.

- Massage, erotic touch.

- Telephone sex (talking with someone about sex on the telephone).
- Fantasy, reading or writing erotic stories.
- Watching someone else touch themselves sexually.
- Sexual intercourse using a latex condom or latex barrier (some risk involved because the condom/barrier might break or slip off).

If neither partner is infected with HIV, the passage of blood, semen or vaginal fluids would not carry an HIV risk. The problem is that many people with HIV feel perfectly well and do not know they are infected, although they can transmit the disease.

Can a person become infected with HIV after just one unsafe experience?
Yes. In most cases of sexual transmission or the sharing of needles, people have experienced multiple exposures to HIV before becoming infected. However, there are some cases where a person has become infected after only one unsafe encounter.

Do condoms prevent HIV?
Yes. Latex condoms, properly used, can provide an effective barrier to HIV.

There are instances where condoms break or slip off. In most cases, these problems are related to "user error." People who are more experienced in the use of condoms are less likely to have problems with breakage and slippage.

What is a latex barrier or latex dam?
A latex barrier is any flat piece of latex that can be used as a barrier during oral-vaginal or oral-anal sex. A latex dam is a square of latex about 6 inches on a side, manufactured for use in dental procedures. You can also make a flat latex barrier by "cutting down" a nonlubricated latex condom. (Make a cut along the length of the condom and cut off the tip, so it can be rolled out flat.)

The flat latex can be placed over the vulva or anus, providing an HIV-resistant barrier for oral sex. No scientific studies have looked at the efficacy of latex barriers in HIV prevention. However, studies have shown that latex condoms are an effective barrier to HIV, and it seems reasonable to believe a "cut down" condom, properly used, will also be effective.

Do sexual lubricants help prevent transmission of HIV?
Lubricants can be helpful in condom use. Properly applied, they can increase the sensation of both partners and decrease incidents of breakage. The lubricant *must* be water-based and water soluble. Any lubricant containing fats or oils (including Crisco, vegetable oil, Vaseline and some commercial sexual lubricants) will break down a latex condom in a matter of seconds.

Some lubricants include spermicides which kill viruses. A common spermicide of this type is nonoxynol-9. A lubricant with nonoxynol-9 may act as a "back up" in case a condom breaks during vaginal or anal intercourse.

However, some individuals have allergic reactions to nonoxynol-9. A rash in the vagina or anus or on the penis would actually increase the risk of HIV infection because it's easier for the virus to pass through breaks in the skin. Before using any lubricants with nonoxynol-9 for sexual purposes, people should test the lubricant by rubbing a little on the inside of the arm over a period of several days. If a rash develops, a person should not use the lubricant.

HIV and Drug Use

What is the correct way to clean needles?
The best way to avoid transmission of HIV through needle use is not to use needles at all. If needles are used, it is safest to never share needles or equipment.

If equipment is shared, cleaning it thoroughly before and after each use can decrease the risk.

For syringes, draw water into the syringe, then expel into the sink or gutter, 3 times. Then draw full-strength bleach into the syringe, and expel into the sink or gutter, 3 times. Keep syringe full of bleach at least 30 seconds each time. Draw water into the syringe again and expel into the sink or gutter, 3 times.

What do alcohol and noninjection drugs have to do with HIV risk?
People are more likely to do things under the influence of drugs or alcohol that they would not otherwise do. Alcohol and most drugs also affect judgment and fine motor coordination.

Under the influence of alcohol or drugs, a person might not follow through on a commitment to follow safer sex guidelines or maintain a monogamous relationship. The fine motor impairment can also make it difficult to use a condom or latex barrier correctly.

In some studies, alcohol has been the substance most commonly associated with the practice of risky sexual behaviors.

Treatment

Will everyone with HIV die?
Over time, the immune systems of most people with HIV become impaired. They experience health problems of increasing severity, usually beginning with mild to moderate illness after 5 to 10 years of infection, with serious and life-threatening episodes after this.

However, researchers in the United States and Europe are now following several hundred individuals who have had HIV infection for 10 or more years and continue to be very healthy. Some of these "long-term survivors" show laboratory signs of immune system decline but continue to be physically sound. Others show little or no sign of immune system damage even after a decade of infection. Studies of these people may provide clues to successful treatment strategies. One day, medical treatments may be able to stop the progression of HIV, making HIV a manageable disease like diabetes or heart disease.

It does not seem to be scientifically accurate or psychologically productive to refer to HIV as a universally fatal disease.

It is more useful to think of HIV as a "life-threatening condition." This respects those living with HIV today and helps everyone look forward to the day that people with HIV will survive the infection.

When will there be a vaccine for HIV?

Vaccine research on HIV has been active for many years, and several vaccines are currently being tested in human trials. An HIV vaccine represents a particular challenge to scientists. So far, there has never been a successful vaccine for a human retrovirus.

Any HIV vaccines that seem promising in initial studies will need to go through a long period of testing before becoming generally available. It is likely that it will be many years before a vaccine is able to be offered. At the present time, prevention is the only "vaccine" we have, and the only one we can count on for the future.

What treatments are available for HIV? When will there be a cure?

A number of medications have been developed that slow progression of HIV. There are also treatments that can help prevent some of the common illnesses that develop in people with HIV. And there are better treatments for many HIV-associated illnesses once they do develop.

Some people with HIV also use non-Western and nonmedical approaches to address their infection. Acupuncture, herbal and Chinese medicine, homeopathy, visualization, vitamins and support groups have all been used, sometimes along with traditional Western medicine.

None of these developments represents a "cure," however. A true cure for HIV is certainly many years away, if it is even possible. Our hope is that the treatments will continue to improve, providing better protection for people with HIV and causing fewer side effects, until HIV becomes a manageable condition.

Testing for HIV

What is the HIV antibody test?

The HIV antibody test is a simple blood test that indicates whether an individual has produced antibodies to HIV.

If the antibody test result is *positive*, it means that antibodies to HIV were detected, and the individual has HIV infection. This person would be capable of transmitting the virus to others during unsafe sexual activities or needle sharing.

If the antibody test result is *negative*, it means that no antibodies to HIV were detected. Either the person is not infected with HIV, or the person is infected but has not yet developed antibodies.

What is the "window period"?

Any time a person is infected with a virus, there is a lag between the infection and the development of antibodies to the virus. This is called the "window period." The window period for development of HIV antibody is usually between 2 weeks and 6 months. Rarely, it might be longer.

If an individual has tested negative on the HIV antibody test, but has had some HIV-related risk within the past 6 months, it would be best to be tested again 6 months after any risky behavior to be confident of the results.

If antibodies protect us from disease, why do people with antibodies to HIV get sick?
Antibodies are specialized proteins produced by the immune system to fight diseases. Some antibodies are fully effective. Most people, for example, have measles only one time in their lives. Their bodies produced antibodies which prevented any future infection of that type. But antibodies to HIV are only partially effective. They seem able to fight progression of the disease at the outset, but appear to lose their effectiveness after a period of time.

Children and HIV

Is the HIV antibody test performed on children?
The HIV antibody test can be performed on children. For newborns of infected mothers, however, the test results are complicated by the presence of maternal antibody in the infant's blood. This means that an infant who tests positive may *not* actually be infected with the virus, but might have antibodies from the mother's blood in its system. This situation usually resolves by the time the child is about 18 months old. The mother's antibodies will have cleared from the child's system by that time. Antibody tests after that will be about as reliable as tests on adults.

There are several other types of tests (including viral cultures and PCR—polymerase chain reaction) that can be performed on infants to determine whether the child has HIV infection. Today, medical providers can usually determine a child's HIV status accurately by about 6 months of age.

How many children have been diagnosed with AIDS?
How did they become infected?
At the end of 1994, about 6,200 children under age 13 had been diagnosed with AIDS. The great majority of these were children of mothers with HIV (about 89%). Smaller numbers of children were infected through the use of medicines treating hemophilia (4%), through blood transfusions (6%), or had an undetermined risk (1%).

Children with AIDS may have carried HIV infection for many years before receiving an AIDS diagnosis. This is why we continue to see some new cases of AIDS associated with use of hemophilia medicines or blood transfusions. However, new cases of HIV infection are now almost solely related to the presence of HIV infection in the mother. Transfusion-associated HIV is very rare today, and medicines used to treat hemophilia no longer carry a risk of HIV infection.

Does HIV affect children the same way it affects adults?
Adults with HIV usually look and feel healthy for many years after first becoming infected. Over time, they begin to develop a number of unusual diseases that are not seen in people with healthy

immune systems, or they develop unusually severe cases of more common diseases.

Children born with HIV tend to follow one of two common profiles of disease progression. In the first, the children develop some of the unusual infections seen in adults with immune system problems. They may also develop unusually severe cases of common childhood illnesses.

In the second, the children do well for many years. Like adults with HIV infection, their immune systems seem able to hold the disease in check for a considerable period of time. Some of these children have lived to age 10 and beyond without serious health problems.

While most children with HIV are still expected to have shortened lifespans complicated by severe illness, it is encouraging to know that some have reached early adolescence in relatively good health.

How serious is the threat of HIV infection of children as a result of sexual molestation?

Any child who is sexually molested faces a number of potential medical and psychological complications. If the perpetrator is infected with HIV, these include the risk of HIV transmission. A number of children have been identified who contracted HIV infection through sexual molestation.

The same behaviors that put adults at risk for HIV—unprotected oral, vaginal or anal intercourse, or passage of blood—also put children at risk. The background risks for perpetrators vary, but may include sharing needles for injection drug use or male-to-male sexual contact.

Teachers, parents and the larger community should be alert to *all* cases of child molestation and the many potential risks involved, and act swiftly to intervene in cases of known or suspected sexual abuse.

How many children with HIV will be attending elementary school?

This is another question that is difficult to answer. While we can count cases of AIDS among elementary-age children (AIDS cases must be reported to departments of health), we do not have a way of counting children with HIV.

It has been estimated that there may be as many as 20,000 to 30,000 children with HIV in the United States today. If these numbers are accurate, most of these children will be perinatal cases infected during pregnancy or at the time of birth. Many children born with HIV will not survive to school age.

However, with earlier identification of HIV infection and better treatments, children with HIV are living longer. Others do not seem to be developing serious illnesses. We suggest that schools prepare themselves for the probability that children with HIV may be attending classes now or in the future.

Aren't most children with HIV the offspring of injection-drug-using parents? Do we have children like that in our school?

Drug use and abuse, including injection drug use, is present in all communities.

Injection drug users may live on the streets, surviving from fix to fix, supporting their habit through criminal activity. But most injection drug users are working people who live in homes and have families.

Even people who only use injection drugs on occasion usually share needles with others at some point. They are likely to see their drug use as "recreational" and not consider it a problem. Since injection drug use is an illegal activity, users are not easy to identify. Denial—of drug dependence and HIV risk—is common and powerful among this population.

Women who do not use injection drugs themselves may become infected through unsafe sex with men who do. In many cases, women infected through unprotected intercourse with a man have no idea how their partners acquired HIV. Although many people are not aware of a significant presence of injection drug users in their communities, the risk of HIV infection through this means is very real.

What is the likelihood of children with HIV passing it to others at school or in community programs?

HIV transmission can only take place when a person takes the blood, semen or vaginal fluids of another person infected with HIV into his or her body. Children are not likely to have this kind of exposure to others in school or community settings.

People often express concerns about a child with HIV fighting with other children or having open sores. If a child with HIV has significant behavioral problems, or has open sores or lesions which cannot be covered, it may be necessary to keep the child from some school activities. This would be an exceptional case. Most children with HIV will do well in a school or community setting and do not pose any risk to their peers.

It is reasonable to be concerned about the presence of blood if a child with HIV is injured. Children should be taught not to touch someone else's blood in the case of an injury, but to call an adult for help.

Teachers and others who work with children should be familiar with proper precautions for first aid and cleaning of body fluid spills. Uniform guidelines for such tasks should be established at all schools and agencies. Latex gloves should be used in response to first-aid situations involving blood. Spills of blood should be cleaned with a 1:10 solution of bleach (1 part bleach to 10 parts water), and vinyl or latex gloves should be worn for cleaning. Hands should be washed with soap and water after first aid or cleaning.

These guidelines will prevent transmission of HIV and many other diseases.

Doubts About Casual Transmission

How can we be sure HIV can't be transmitted casually?

People often have this understandable concern. HIV is a serious, life-threatening disease. New information is being reported on HIV and AIDS all the time. Government and civic officials often discount worries about casual transmission, but some people do not trust these reassurances.

However, we actually know a great deal about HIV. We know quite a bit about its structure. We understand how the virus attacks the immune system, and we have seen that it is fragile and dies quickly outside the human body. We are also familiar now with the progression of disease and the range of illnesses that affect people with HIV.

From studies of thousands of people, we understand that HIV is transmitted only in certain circumstances—most often where blood, semen or vaginal fluids of an infected person enter the body of someone else. There are also some medical situations where the blood, organs or internal body fluids of an infected person have entered the body of someone else and infection has developed.

The information about HIV transmission and prevention has not changed significantly since the mid-1980s. Most of the new information reported today either refines what we already know about HIV or addresses issues for which we do not yet have answers: how to stop the progression of disease, how to cure it, how to vaccinate against it, and how to get people to follow prevention guidelines.

People's questions about casual transmission are likely to continue. But a close look at the most common questions reinforces the scientific findings that HIV is not casually transmitted.

Could people who have had casual contact with someone with AIDS be in the incubation period? Couldn't the disease appear years from now?
The incubation period for AIDS is the span of time between first infection with HIV and the development of signs or symptoms which qualify for an AIDS diagnosis. It may be 10 years or longer in some individuals. This is a long time.

However, the length of time between first infection and development of HIV antibodies is fairly short, usually in 2 to 12 weeks and occasionally taking as long as 6 months. It is easy to test for the presence of HIV antibody. If someone had been infected through casual contact, evidence would be available within a short period of time.

Many antibody studies have been performed on family members of people with HIV who share casual contact, and there has never been a spread of infection except where there is a known risk activity—for example, if a man and woman have unprotected sexual intercourse. There have also been studies of residential school settings where some students were known to have HIV. In dozens of such studies carried out worldwide, there has never been evidence of transmission through casual contact.

Couldn't the AIDS cases in the United States that are classified as "Other/Risk Not Reported or Identified" have been transmitted through casual contact?
Reporting on a disease diagnosed in over 500,000 Americans is a true challenge. Those affected are dispersed over the entire country and are treated in a variety of medical settings. Yet, of these hundreds of thousands of individuals, 94% have an established, common risk factor.

Of the remaining 6%, a certain number involve unusual risks, such as health care providers or laboratory workers exposed in work settings. One person was infected after intentional self-inoculation with HIV-infected blood. A few adolescents who acquired HIV perinatally were not diagnosed with AIDS until after age 13. All of these individuals are included in the "Other" category.

Early in the epidemic, a few thousand people were placed in the "heterosexual transmission" category because they came from areas with high prevalence of HIV, like Haiti or Africa. In retrospect, the Centers for Disease Control and Prevention (CDC), who tabulates this data, acknowledged that some of these individuals might have also been infected through shared needles or male-to-male sex. Since information on these older cases is very limited, most have had to be labeled as "Risk Not Identified."

The CDC places all AIDS cases under active investigation into this category. On careful follow-up by local public health officials, most cases initially entered as "risk not identified" are found to have well-established or suspected risk factors. Once the risk factors become clear, the case is moved to the proper category.

However, in some cases, further information does not become available. The reasons the CDC cannot establish risk factors for some individuals include:

1. The most common risk factors for HIV—sharing injection drug equipment or having unsafe, male-to-male sexual contact—are highly stigmatized activities. Many people are unable or unwilling to admit to these behaviors.

2. Some people visit a medical facility when they are ill and do not return for later follow-up. Diagnostic tests run at the initial visit may result in a diagnosis of AIDS at a later time. Because the individual does not return, no further information can be gathered on the person's risk history.

3. Some people are too ill at the time of an AIDS diagnosis to provide information about themselves.

4. Some individuals are diagnosed with AIDS after death. Risk information is often unavailable in these circumstances.

Years of careful follow-up by highly skilled epidemiologists has not always led to absolute answers about the risk factors for every case of AIDS, but there has never been evidence in any of these investigations of casual transmission of HIV.

Further Information

Where can I get answers to questions not answered here?

You can get questions about HIV answered through the toll-free National AIDS Hotline.

English: (800) 342-AIDS (or 342-2437)

Spanish: (800) 344-SIDA (or 344-7432)

Deaf Access: (800) 243-7889 (TTD/TTY)

There are also local resources that can provide you with further information. The National AIDS Hotline can tell you about information resources in your area.

What Can Children Understand, When?

THOUGH THEORISTS IN THE PAST have believed that children were essentially "stuck" at a particular cognitive level of development based on their chronological age, more recent research shows that this is only partially true. While children do, appropriately, have limitations in their ability to process very complex information, they are also capable of increasing to some extent their capacity to understand more abstract concepts. For the most part, given the opportunity, children can accomplish more sophisticated learning than was once believed.

General statements are often made about what children can understand at different ages, but teachers often see wide variations from child to child and classroom to classroom. Each class and each child have unique characteristics and experiences that influence learning and styles of thinking. In fact, many teachers of middle and high school students describe students who habitually employ thinking styles associated with younger children, while some elementary teachers have seen young students apply surprisingly sophisticated reasoning to a subject or lesson.

Teachers may find it more helpful to develop an understanding of the broader sequence of learning in different subject areas. Then, regardless of the chronological age of the child, the teacher can provide classroom experiences that help solidify learning at the present developmental stage and offer opportunities to move along in the developmental sequence.

Health and Illness

Children typically move through a series of stages in understanding the causes of illness. The explanations of very young children tend to be *egocentric* and employ *magical thinking*—they feel involved in and responsible for the things that happen around them. Illness is seen as a form of punishment for either real or imagined wrong-doing: "I misbehaved at dinner, and that night my little brother got sick and had to go to the hospital." Older children and even adults may have some of these same concerns and beliefs when serious illness or death occurs in someone important to them.

When asked how a person gets sick, children at this stage often provide circular responses. For example, a child might explain that, "You get AIDS by getting sick." They also use *phenomenistic* responses—that is, the child refers to some phenomenon, or aspect, of an illness as if it were the cause. "You catch a cold by getting a runny nose," a child explains. "You get pneumonia by not being able to breathe." Children at this stage may assign the cause of many events to benign or unrelated occurrences—often just because the events occurred about the same time. "The electricity went off in our house last night and we had to light candles, and this morning I woke up with a cold."

Often as early as preschool, children begin to develop a more accurate understanding of physical illness. They understand that illnesses have causes, that germs play a role, and that people can contract illnesses from one another. However, they often fail to make the distinction between communicable and non-communicable diseases and may overgeneralize concerns about disease transmission to non-contagious illnesses as well. Children may fear catching diseases like cancer or conditions that have required hospitalization among family members, friends or public figures, such as heart disease or diabetes.

Children at this stage also retain very concrete notions about how germs operate in the world. "A cold germ can get into the body," suggests to some children that illnesses are caused by a solitary germ, and that it roams around alone inside the body. They are told to cover their mouths when coughing so they will not "give" their cold to someone else. But if they want to get rid of a cold, it seems like a good idea to leave the mouth uncovered so they can try to give it away.

Juxtapositions that would seem mutually exclusive to most adults can coexist comfortably in the minds of many young children. This is why it is not surprising to hear a child claim that the AIDS germ lives in blood, and that AIDS is caused by drugs; or that most people in the world already have AIDS, even though she or he knows few people who do. Children's explanations continue to be generalized and nonspecific.

As children mature, they are able to provide *concrete, specific causes* of an illness. These might be accurate or inaccurate. For example, a child might explain that a person can catch a cold "from a germ" (accurate), or "from going outside without a coat on" (inaccurate). However, they cannot yet explain how illness results from these acts or from contact with these agents. They may be able to tell you that people catch colds from viruses, but have no understanding of how contact is made with the virus or how illness results once contact has been made.

For children to progress to the next stage of understanding of health and illness, they must appreciate that a *disease-causing agent must enter or act on the body* in a particular manner. At this stage, children might explain, "If you get too much sunlight on your skin, then you can get cancer." They may still confuse the facts they have about various illnesses, however, blending explanations for communicable and non-communicable illnesses ("A person catches leukemia when someone coughs on them").

An essential foundation for further advancement is the ability to differentiate between separate diseases. Once children thoroughly understand that each disease is unique, and that diseases vary in their causes, symptoms, treatments and outcomes, they are able to absorb an impressive amount of distinct data about different illnesses. At a more advanced stage of understanding illness, children can identify the *specific effect of the disease-causing agent* ("The AIDS virus gets into your body and kills your white blood cells"), while the final stage involves an appreciation of the *underlying causes and process of disease* ("When your white blood cells don't work, you can't fight off other sicknesses and you get sick.")

Death

Many teachers are apprehensive about discussing death in the classroom, and these concerns may emerge when AIDS education is proposed. It is important to be prepared for a range of comments and questions from young students who are learning about AIDS, and some of these might well involve death and dying. However, the lessons in this curriculum are not about death, but about health, illness and communicable disease. In the framework in which the material is presented, death is less likely to become a major focus.

Like many other complex subjects, children's information about death is often incorrect. In movies, television shows, video games and children's stories, references to death are common but confusing. In some cases, characters die and then come back to life. In others, people who die continue to appear as ghostlike phantoms or very solid figures, their bodies vigorous and active, their involvement with the living extensive. Causes of death may seem magical, determined by fate or destiny. And clever heroes in all of these media are able to overcome the most extraordinary obstacles, escaping death in spite of bullets, automobile accidents, freezing temperatures, lethal poisons or any number of other dangers.

We may not be able to answer all of children's questions about death, but we can provide them with some of the most basic concepts as a foundation for more realistic and reassuring understandings. These include:

- Death is irreversible.
- All life functions cease completely at the time of death.
- There are true causes why living things die.
- Death is inevitable.

At very early ages, children's views of death, like other ways they see the world, are often constructed through magical and egocentric thinking. Children may therefore feel responsible for loss or death, as they might for an episode of illness in a family member or friend. They often have not been told, or do not understand, the real reasons why people die. They may also believe that death is avoidable or reversible.

In addition, young children may think that inanimate objects, such as dolls or stuffed toys, are alive. They may not understand all the physical differences between life and death and may therefore worry that a dead relative is still hungry or in pain.

As children grow older, often around the ages of 6 to 8, they are better able to see death as a final and inevitable outcome for all living things. Like many adults, however, the concept of their own death may be more problematic. It is hard to accept that one's experience of the physical world could end. During this period, children are often very interested in the physical details of death. Adults may find their fascination with coffins, funerals or what dead things look or smell like perplexing. It is out of their great curiosity about the world around them, however, that children pursue these interests with such zeal. It is also around this age that children often develop a concern for spiritual and religious matters: what happens to the soul after the body dies.

The section Talking with Children About Death (p. 193) reviews this topic in greater detail.

Reproduction*

Children also follow a predictable sequence in developing their understanding of reproduction. As in other subject areas, adults can offer "correct" explanations for things, but children who do not have the conceptual basis to understand a factual explanation are likely to continue to develop theories more consistent with what they already know. Adult theories often simply do not make sense to children in the context of their own experiences.

Preschool-age children are just beginning to cope with information that is abstract in nature. Their skills in mastering abstract concepts are limited, however, and their explanations for events are likely to be fairly concrete. For example, a child seeing a visibly pregnant woman guesses that the woman has eaten something to make her stomach fat. If the child understands that there is a baby developing inside the woman, he or she might believe that the baby first existed someplace else, and was then magically placed inside the mother's body.

Anne Bernstein, a researcher who explored how children of different ages understood information about reproduction and birth, called children in this age group "the geographers," because their theories focus on where the baby has come from (the store, the hospital, the mother's tummy). Geographers believe the baby has always existed and for some reason has now come to live in their family.

At the next stage of understanding, children guess that babies are manufactured by people in the same way cars are produced in a factory. "Manufacturers" create stories to explain how the baby was made: the mother ate something that

---

*This section is adapted from *When Sex Is the Subject: Attitudes and Answers for Young Children.* P. M. Wilson. 1991. Santa Cruz, CA: ETR Associates.

grew inside her tummy. When children hear language like, "the father plants his seed in the mother," this further confirms this type of mythical thinking.

The early elementary years are a time of enormous cognitive growth for children, and they continue to move towards increasingly abstract thinking. By age 6 or 7, most children are beginning to understand generalizations that go beyond their concrete experiences. Their ideas are starting to be strongly influenced not only by what they see and hear but by what they read.

Bernstein sees this stage as a transitional period in a child's understanding of reproduction. Children in this age group may be able to recite the basic facts about reproduction, but they do not quite grasp the full story. Maybe they know the mother's egg meets with the father's sperm, but they think the egg is large and has a shell. They may know that it takes a man and a woman to make a baby, but perhaps they think the man and woman have to be married for reproduction to occur.

During later elementary years—ages 9 to 12—children are increasingly ready to be challenged in their literal styles of thinking. They are open to new information. While they may not automatically think deeply about new ideas, they do respond well to opportunities to reflect in more abstract ways on information they are learning.

Bernstein labels the next levels of children's understanding "concrete physiology" and "preformation." Concrete physiologists can consider past, present and future, and understand cause and effect. It is clear to them that sexual intercourse is the vehicle for bringing together the sperm and the egg, but they are not sure why it is necessary for these cells to unite. Children who believe in preformation think the fetus already exists in either the sperm or the egg, and that the connection between these cells is only needed to promote the growth of the pre-existing fetus. It is not until around age 12 that most children can really put the story of reproduction together completely.

Sexuality

As children are going through this sequence of understanding about reproduction, they are also being exposed to a wide range of information and experience about sexuality. Most elementary-age children engage in some forms of sex play and masturbation. They are clear on gender distinctions (that boys and girls are biologically different), and they have attached themselves to sex-role behaviors (boys act in one way, girls in another). Even young children have often gained rather sophisticated data about adult sexuality through news broadcasts, family discussions, magazines, movies, MTV and "adult" cable channels.

In the same way that children apply concrete explanations to reproductive processes that baffle them, they are likely to develop mythical theories about the purposes and drives behind adult sexuality. There has been surprisingly little research in this area, however. We do not really know what children understand about sex except as it relates to reproduction. We do know, from studies of children's understanding about reproduction, that where accurate answers are not available, children will construct their own explanations. And these are often very creative but far from accurate.

Studies of children's concepts about sexual behavior in relation to reproduction do reveal that the use of analogies to explain biological processes is confusing to children. They tend to understand these allusions in very concrete and literal terms. Adult's analogies have generated children's descriptions of "eggs" in the mother encased in firm, brittle shells, looking something like chicken eggs, or explanations that fathers purchase special seed packets at stores and plant these in soil in the mother's stomach, watering them on occasion with semen.

Because our sense of children's understanding of sexual drives and attractions remains incomplete, guidelines for classroom discussion are more general than for other topics in this area. There are no defined stages to help children advance through. There is, however, a clear imperative to provide children with honest and accurate answers at an appropriate level of thoroughness. In some cases, teachers may be able to provide this information directly. In others, referral to parents or other resources may be necessary. In all events, it is most useful to offer children information as they request it, in a format that gently challenges the concrete, mythical or egocentric beliefs they are likely to hold concerning adult sexuality.

Guidelines for Discussing Sensitive Topics

YOU MAY FIND YOURSELF in a special kind of bind when providing AIDS education in an elementary classroom. If your teaching is interesting and involving, students will participate actively and demonstrate their interest by asking many questions. It is likely they will ask questions about topics that are sensitive or controversial, such as sexuality, substance use and death. Most of these will be good questions, deserving of accurate and informed answers.

However, many schools and districts have policies prohibiting explicit discussion of such topics in classrooms. In a number of schools, teachers are not allowed to say certain words, such as *homosexual* or *condom*. Even if they have considerable freedom about how they handle a topic like AIDS, teachers may feel apprehensive about their ability to discuss complex and value-laden topics like sexuality, substance use or death. They may worry they do not have the necessary information to answer accurately, the necessary background to answer sensitively, or the confidence to address the material in a way that is reassuring and helpful to students.

The positive side of this dilemma is that, as an elementary-level teacher, you already have extensive expertise in discussing "sensitive" issues with your students. Young children do not make the same kinds of distinctions adults do about the sensitivity of different kinds of information. A question about why one student can run faster than another may feel just as "sensitive" to a first grader as a question about how a woman gets pregnant or why people have sex.

Answering Students' Questions

The same kinds of skills you use in any discussion with your students will be useful in discussions about sensitive topics, with a few additional recommendations based on the possibility of school policies or outside controversy. The following guidelines offer a step-by-step approach to answering children's questions about sensitive subjects.

Consider the intent behind the question. When children ask a question, their actual intent may not be immediately apparent. Consider what the child wants to find out before providing your answer. The child may be seeking information, expressing anxiety, or testing out solutions to problems. In some cases, the child is seeking some kind of reaction by asking a question known to be difficult or embarrassing. Frame your response based on your best understanding of what the child really wants.

Answer directly and validate the child's interest. When a sensitive topic is raised, offer a response that directly acknowledges the importance of the subject matter and confirms the appropriateness of the child's interest in the material. Let students know that you are listening to them.

A direct answer is not necessarily the same thing as a complete answer. For example, if a child asks an explicit question about sex and you are in a school that does not allow teachers to discuss sexuality in classrooms, you can acknowledge this in your answer.

Answer honestly and avoid using euphemisms. Because children's thinking is often magical (things occur through mysterious powers) or mythical (explanations are not based on actual facts), it is important to offer factual information that can clear up misconceptions. While it is not desirable to force children to give up magical thinking styles entirely, it is helpful for them to be exposed to a variety of possible explanations for events around them, including those based on fact.

In situations where misconceptions are causing unnecessary guilt or anxiety, children need to be provided with a more accurate understanding. Teachers who provide this reassurance establish a foundation of trust that can be of great value to children, and enables them to move into more sophisticated conceptual stages as they are ready.

Provide appropriate reassurance. Many points of information about AIDS can raise anxiety for children. Teachers who recognize and anticipate this can build reassurances into their discussions. For example, "AIDS is a very serious disease. Fortunately, it is not a disease that affects children your age very often, so the students in this class do not need to worry about catching AIDS."

Acknowledge limitations. There are any number of limitations that can arise for teachers addressing AIDS in the classroom. Perhaps most common among these are knowledge (the teacher does not know the answer to a question), school policies (the teacher is not allowed to discuss a particular topic with students), or the needs and understanding of other students (other students may not understand the nature of the question or might be less interested in the details, or the question might be more sophisticated than necessary for most of the class).

In all of these cases, it is important to acknowledge the limitations directly and honestly. Along with this, provide guidance for students that will give them some possibilities for satisfying their curiosity. For example, a teacher who does not know an answer can offer to research the material and come back with more information later on. A student who raises a topic that cannot be discussed in the classroom because of school policies can be referred to his or her parents. A student who has asked a question that will be of little benefit to the rest of the class can be invited to discuss the matter individually with the teacher during recess or at some other time.

Refer to parents or other sources as necessary. If parents have been notified ahead of time that AIDS will be addressed in the curriculum, they will be better prepared for questions from their children. Value-related questions, such as the morality of using drugs, the purpose of sexuality, or the nature of the soul can be referred back to parents when they arise.

Avoid answers that might cause students to feel badly about family members. Remember that some students may have parents or other family members who drink alcohol, smoke or use other drugs; have sex outside of marriage; are in primary relationships without being married; are divorced; are gay or lesbian; or do not believe in God. Phrase your answers in a nonjudgmental fashion, so that children do not feel conflicted, embarrassed or alienated from the class or their families. For example, avoid describing people who use drugs as "bad," or suggesting that someone who does not stay in a committed, lifelong monogamous relationship is morally wrong.

Monitor the sharing of personal information by students and prevent inappropriate personal disclosures. Children are usually eager to discuss topics like AIDS and sexuality with caring and supportive adults, and may disclose information inappropriate for the general classroom setting ("My father does cocaine and gets high every night." "My cousin Susie has AIDS and my dad said she got it from doing drugs."). You will need to monitor the degree to which students share personal information to help prevent inappropriate personal disclosures.

Teachers know their students well, and can often sense when they are about to disclose information. By responding promptly and redirecting the question, such disclosures can often be halted early on ("Yes, people can get AIDS from using drugs. Can anyone explain what we learned about how this happens?"). Be sure to speak with the child during the next class break and explain why you did not respond directly to the question asked. You can also offer support and assistance if this seems appropriate.

One way to lower the frequency of these situations is to suggest to the class that private matters be discussed with their parents or in individual discussions with you. "Most children your age do not need to be worried about having AIDS. But if any of you are worried about whether you or someone you care about may have AIDS, you can speak with your parents. I would also be happy to speak with you about this individually, after class." Avoid asking children directly about personal experiences when their answers might lead to inappropriate disclosures.

Be reliable about follow-up. If you say you will research something you do not know about, or bring in a resource that can explain something further, be sure to do so in a timely fashion.

Examples of How to Handle Sensitive Topics

Each classroom situation will present its own unique circumstances, but it may be useful to look over some of the comments and statements other teachers have made when addressing sensitive issues in the classroom.

School Policies Prohibiting Explicit Discussions About Sexuality

In these situations, it is generally most helpful to validate the question, acknowledge the school policy, and provide an alternate resource from which the child can obtain an answer. Referrals back to parents or an invitation to talk privately are especially helpful.

- **"What do people do when they have 'close sexual contact'?"**

    "We've used the term 'close sexual contact' in this class several times. I think it's important for you to get answers to your questions, but the school has asked that we not talk about sex in class. Because your question is important, I suggest you ask your parents about it tonight. Your parents know we are talking about this in class, and should be happy to answer any questions you might have. Let me know tomorrow if they were able to answer your questions."

- **"Would people catch AIDS if someone's condom breaks while they're having sex?"**

    "This is a good question, and an important one to get answered. But the school has asked that we not talk about condoms in this classroom. I'd like to suggest you talk with your parents about this question. They know we are talking about AIDS in class, and I think they'll be happy to answer your question. Or, if you'd prefer, you can also talk with me privately during the break and I can talk with you more about your question then."

Philosophical or Moral Questions

Because students' families probably have a range of philosophical and moral beliefs, it is most appropriate for teachers to avoid firm pronouncements on these issues. Instead, again validate the question, acknowledge that it is a question about values, and refer students to their families for further discussion.

- **"When you die, don't you go to heaven and live with God?"**

    "We know that the activities of the body—eating, breathing, feeling pain—end when someone dies. But no one knows for sure what else happens to a person when he or she dies. Some people believe in a special place called heaven, and believe God lives there with the souls of people who have died. This is a good question to talk over with your parents

How AIDS Works: Grades K–3

and other people in your family. There are many different beliefs about what happens to people after they die."

- **"Are people who use drugs bad?"**

    "I do not think that people who use drugs are bad, but I know that using drugs can be a bad thing. Some of you may have done something that got you into trouble at some time. This doesn't mean you are a bad person, but it might mean you did something that was not a good thing to do.

    "People who use drugs frequently and cannot stop using them do not want to hurt themselves or other people, but often they do not know how to stop using drugs. Most have tried to stop many times.

    "This is one reason we try so hard to keep students like you from getting involved with drugs in the first place. Once drug use becomes a problem, it is very hard for a person to stop."

- **"Are people who have sex without being married bad?"**

    "This is a question that can be answered in many different ways. Different people have different beliefs about sex, and that includes what they believe about having sex without being married.

    "This is a good question to talk over with your parents and other people in your family. You can think about how you feel about this question when you understand more about the things they believe."

Questions Too Sophisticated for the Class

Sometimes a student asks questions that are much more sophisticated than those of the rest of the class. For example, one first grader asks explicit questions about condoms falling off while other students are asking one another what a condom is.

Teachers need not provide explicit detail regarding sexuality for the benefit of a few precocious students. It is always helpful to affirm the importance of a student's questions, but in many cases it will be most appropriate to redirect a student to private discussion after class, or to alternate sources of information, especially parents.

- **"What is a guy supposed to do if he can't use a condom because he can't keep his penis hard?"**

    "You have asked a good question, but it is also a complicated one. I think this is something I could explain more easily if we talk about it privately after class. You could also ask your parents about this, and I think they would be able to give you a good answer."

Questions Using Explicit or Slang Terms

When students use slang terms, especially if these are offensive, you can rephrase the question using more conventional language. It is important to do this in a matter-of-fact way, without seeming to judge or correct the student. In many children's families, these kinds of slang terms are part of everyday language, and this may be the clearest way the student can articulate the question.

- **"Can people get AIDS from sucking tits?"**

    "This question—whether people can get the AIDS germ from nipples or breasts—is a good one. Most of the time, people cannot get AIDS from nipples or breasts. However, if a mother has the AIDS germ and breastfeeds her baby, the baby might get the germ through the breast milk."

Questions About Sexual Orientation

Because AIDS has affected gay men in large numbers, discussions of AIDS both in and out of the classroom often bring up questions about homosexuality and sexual orientation. Children deserve straightforward and direct answers to their questions about sexual orientation. Teachers will also want to avoid making judgments about gay and lesbian people. It is important to help children correct misconceptions about HIV transmission that are based on myths and misunderstandings about homosexuality.

- **"What is a homosexual?"**

    "A person who likes to be close to and be sexual with someone of the same sex is called gay, or homosexual. This would be men with men, or women with women. Someone who likes to be close to and be sexual with someone of the opposite sex is called straight, or heterosexual. This would be women with men. Some people like to be close to both men and women; they are called bisexual.

    "These words describe the kind of close, romantic relationships that grown-ups have. They are different from friendships. Children your age, as well as adults, often have very close friendships with same-sex friends. Most boys your age are closest to other boys, and most girls are closest to other girls. This isn't the same thing as being gay."

- **"Do gay people get AIDS because what they do is bad?"**

    "No. People get AIDS because the AIDS germ got into their body. Some people get AIDS from having sex with someone who has the AIDS germ. They might be gay people or heterosexual people. But sex isn't bad, and neither are people who have sex."

- **"Are homosexuals bad?"**

    "No. Homosexuals are just like other kinds of people. Most are good and honest people. A few probably are not.

    "There are people who believe that homosexual behavior is wrong. This is often part of their religious belief. Many other people believe that being gay is just fine. You might want to talk to your parents and family about

How AIDS Works: Grades K–3

what they believe about gay people.

"It is important to remember that in this school, we respect people's right to be who they are. If a teacher or parent is gay, we treat that person with the same respect we have for anyone else."

Fears About Having AIDS

Sometimes, children will express concerns about having AIDS during classroom discussions. Many children are concerned that they might have AIDS or will one day contract it. Because these concerns are so common, teachers are encouraged to provide frequent reassurance to children when discussing AIDS. As noted earlier, teachers can make a general statement to the class before the lesson, reminding the students that most children their age do not need to worry about having AIDS. Students who do have concerns can be encouraged to speak with their parents or to the teacher after class.

Children's fears about having AIDS are usually unfounded, but it is important not to dismiss them out of hand. There will be situations where a child's fears are reasonable. There have been unfortunate incidents where children have contracted HIV through sexual molestation. Children may have also experienced accidental needlesticks on playgrounds where used syringes have been discarded, or in home environments where a family member is receiving medications through injections.

Whenever a child expresses concerns about having AIDS, he or she should be referred to a trustworthy adult who can discuss these matters privately in more detail.

- **"I have a friend who thinks she has AIDS, but she is afraid to tell anyone about it."**

    "I feel that children who are afraid they might have AIDS should tell a grownup they trust—especially their parents—about their fears. Something as important as this is hard even for adults to handle by themselves. If any of you ever had fears like this and did not feel comfortable telling your parents, I hope you would let me know so I could help."

Talking with Children About Death

David J. Schonfeld and Murray Kappelman

DEATH IS A TOPIC most teachers would rather not discuss, let alone teach. It is easy to understand why surveys show that very few elementary school teachers deal with the subject in any planned manner in their classes. Death is an uncomfortable topic to think about, so we look for reasons not to teach it. We rationalize by thinking inwardly, "How can I even begin to explain something to my class of small children that I don't understand well myself?"

What we may fail to realize is how much greater a disadvantage young pupils have when coming to grips with this mystifying reality. They may lack an understanding of even the most basic concepts about what it means when someone they know dies. They are unable, then, to understand what has occurred and to begin to deal with the loss.

Can children learn this type of information without our assistance? Not easily. Parents and other significant adults in their lives (including teachers) often unsuccessfully attempt to protect them from the experience and the knowledge. But what these well-meaning adults fail to grasp is that virtually all children, by the time they reach school age, have had some experience with death that is significant to them. Avoiding the subject in school and at home only creates more mystery and fear.

Do these experiences involve the kinds of losses an adult would appreciate? Not always. One girl, for example, raised her hand in a school assembly to share a significant personal loss story with the group. She had found a spider in her bedroom, and without her family's knowledge, had raised it as a pet, bringing it crumbs to eat and watching it spinning its web. One day a family member found the spider and killed it. As the girl recounted this story, she began to cry. The loss for her was far more significant than her family could have realized. Such "minor" but significant losses occur regularly in children's lives.

Yet the information children are given about death is almost invariably incorrect. Television and children's stories are full of references to death, but typically depict it inaccurately—characters die and later return to life with regularity. Parents and other adults often try and replace deceased pets and give children false assurances, such as telling them that they will never die. It is not surprising, then,

---

Reprinted with permission from *Education Week*, Volume 11, No. 25, March 4, 1992.

that children do not learn these basic facts easily without added guidance. Teachers, in fact, may be their only source of correct information.

We can prepare children for later losses by teaching them this information before they need to use it. As with all topics, we have to teach children information prior to the time it is needed, to allow for mastery and acquisition of skills. If we wait till a child is faced with the death of a close relative or friend, we have waited too long.

Through our work with schools, we have found that teachers who are armed with insight and information feel freer to allow discussions about death to occur in their classrooms. Many, moreover, are pleasantly surprised by how well such instruction is received, and how comfortable the children become with the discussion. We may not be able to answer all of children's questions about death, but we can certainly provide them with some of the most basic concepts as a foundation for their future. These include the following.

Death is irreversible. Children need to understand that death is a permanent phenomenon. There is no return or recovery from death, no matter how much we may wish otherwise. The child who expects the deceased to return, as if he had gone away on a trip, may be angry at the one who has died for not coming back, or even bothering to call. If the child does not appreciate the irreversibility of death, then there is also no reason to begin to detach personal ties to the deceased, a necessary first step in the mourning process.

All life functions cease at the time of death. Children must understand that all of the activities of body and mind—eating, breathing, cognition, sensation, and so on—cease completely at the time of death. Young children who do not understand this may wish to bury pet food with their dead dog, or may be unduly concerned about a deceased relative's being hungry, cold or in pain. They will tell you that dead people don't see well because it is dark underground, or that they can't move "as much" because they are restrained by the coffin.

Failure to understand this concept often leads to a preoccupation with the physical suffering of the dead person. In one assembly of fourth graders, 3 of the children had experienced the death of a parent or guardian in the previous 12 to 18 months. Each had been to a wake where the casket was open and all of them had thought, at some point, that they saw the body move. Because of their incomplete understanding of the concept of death's finality, all 3 children still had recurrent nightmares that their parent or guardian was, in some way, "buried alive," fighting to get out of the grave. Merely explaining the concept to these children helped them by reducing this unnecessary fear—a fear that is unfortunately augmented by some horror movies and sensational stories in supermarket tabloids.

There are true causes why living things die. The child must develop a realistic understanding of the true causes of death. Young children, who lack this understanding, will often reach the conclusion that bad thoughts or unrelated actions (or omissions) were responsible for the death of a loved one. This leads to excessive guilt that is very difficult for the child to resolve. It is almost universal for those close to someone who has died to question whether there was something they did, or failed to do, that was related to the death. But most adults, after considerable introspection, will correctly reach the conclusion that they were not, in fact, responsible. That is because they know the real reason for the death.

Children who lack an understanding of the true causes of death are not able to reach this conclusion; they are left instead with little as an alternative to self-blame. As one bright second grader matter-of-factly stated: "My brother died of sudden infant death syndrome because I went away to camp that day." Only after a discussion of the true causes of death was the boy able to absolve himself of his perceived responsibility for his brother's death.

Death is inevitable. The child must learn that death is a natural phenomenon; every living thing eventually dies. Children who feel that significant individuals, such as themselves or their parents, are immortal are indicating their lack of appreciation of the inevitability of death. Parents and other adults will often question why children need to know "this harsh fact of life" at young ages. What harm, they may argue, is there in protecting their children from this reality for "as long as possible"? The problem is that death is a reality; someone or something of importance to the child will eventually die, and usually before the parent feels it is time to acknowledge this "harsh reality." If the child does not view death as inevitable, then he or she is likely to view death as a form of punishment, either for actions or thoughts of the deceased or of the child. This, in turn, leads to excessive guilt and shame that makes coping and adjustment to the loss very difficult.

Studies have shown that even very young children are capable of understanding these concepts about death. Most children, in fact, learn them between the ages of 5 and 7. Education has been shown to even further advance the understanding of the young child (that is, prekindergarten through second grade). But teachers need not create formal death-education classes in the primary and elementary grades. Instead, we recommend that they make a conscious attempt to integrate information about death into existing curricula, and that they take advantage of spontaneous class discussions and naturally occurring events, such as when a student finds a dead goldfish in the class fish tank or a dead bug on the playground.

Children have many questions about death and are eager to discuss it once the topic has been broached by a caring adult. One child, on hearing that we would be talking about death in her class, pulled out a picture she had drawn earlier that day of an elaborate graveyard scene and was eager to discuss it. Her teacher seemed surprised by the picture, but such drawings are common among young children and need not be cause for alarm. In fact, young children find the topic fascinating.

Teachers also may wish to take advantage of the many excellent stories and videos dealing with death that can be found in the school system or at local libraries. Educational materials should be selected that present the information clearly and accurately and that reinforce the relevant concepts in a manner that is developmentally appropriate for the intended group.

It is reasonable for teachers to be concerned that when they first begin discussing death in their classroom children will challenge them with questions they fear are inappropriate—or perhaps impossible to answer. Questions involving religious beliefs actually occur infrequently in the primary and early-elementary grades. When they do, such questions as "When you die, don't you go to heaven to live with God?" can easily be answered with statements such as "No one knows for sure what happens when someone dies; some people believe in a special place called heaven where they believe God lives." The children can, and should, be directed back to their parents and family if they want further information touching on religious beliefs.

At times children will also ask questions for which no good answer is available, such as "But why did my dog have to die so young? It just isn't fair." Such questions should be answered honestly, reflecting the lack of an adequate explanation.

Older children, in the later elementary grades, may ask questions relating to details of body preparation, burial, and decomposition that may make the teacher initially uncomfortable. In one assembly of fourth graders, several children wanted to know why the eyes remained closed during the wake and funeral. Unsatisfied by simple assurance that the body was prepared so that they would not open, they persisted with this line of inquiry, reflecting their age-appropriate curiosity. Once informed that the eyelids were sewn closed, they moved quickly onto new questions, with little reaction other than a brief, "Oh, gross."

In fact, children of this age group are able to provide much more vivid and unsettling images drawn from their own imaginations and supplemented by exposure to graphic horror films.

Most children will not become upset by these discussions. But for an occasional child, the teacher's willingness to talk about death may provide the opportunity for expressing feelings about prior or current crises, some related to death, some not. Children have used these occasions, for example, to talk about their concerns regarding their parent's drug abuse, ongoing physical abuse in the home, or unresolved feelings about prior losses. Teachers will need to be prepared to deal with such situations when they arise, and they should know about appropriate resources for children within their school and community.

Teachers must remember that the

child who is upset during such discussions is invariably expressing feelings and emotions that existed prior to the discussion; the teacher's willingness to "hear" these feelings is the reason that the child is able to express them. The discussion did not cause the upset, but only allowed its expression, a needed first step toward its resolution.

The intensity of the discussions should be monitored, however, and when it seems appropriate the conversation should be refocused on positive coping techniques (such as talking to people, drawing pictures) and on sources of support within the home (emphasizing parents), school and community. Children can then raise their hand to share with the group about when their dog died and be asked in turn "What helped you feel better then?" Other students will eagerly volunteer activities that made them feel better when they were sad. An individual student who appears to have more to discuss than is appropriate for the classroom setting can be approached individually after class.

Teachers will be amazed, though, at the capacity of even very young children to tolerate sad emotions in a caring context and to assist their peers. In one second-grade class, a boy began to cry during a film because he was reminded of the death of his pet dog a year earlier. When the film was stopped, the boy insisted on remaining for its conclusion and asked that it be restarted. Without any prompting, a classmate brought him a box of tissues and another child put his arm around the boy's shoulder.

In a prekindergarten class, a girl who had not been present for the class's discussion about death the week before returned from the weekend and told a friend that her grandmother had died. The teacher was proud to overhear the friend offer support and advice on coping techniques: "You could try drawing a picture of your grandmother," the child said. "Sometimes that helps you feel better."

Addressing Drug Use and AIDS

THIS SECTION BRIEFLY OUTLINES how to review issues concerning drug use if students haven't already covered the material. These discussion suggestions are provided with the *strong* recommendation that a separate curriculum address this important topic in more depth.

Background on Drug Use

Provide background on drug use generally, and injection drug use specifically. Younger students may be able to volunteer less information, and you may need to fill in more of the discussion for them. Following are suggested questions to assess students' knowledge of various topics concerning drug use.

- **Students' awareness of drug use**

  Sometimes, older children and adults use drugs. These are not drugs from a doctor, but drugs they buy illegally. Have any of you heard of people doing this?

  Look for affirmative responses.

- **Types of drugs people may use**

  What are some drugs people use?

  Look for responses listing drugs common in the community.

- **Reasons for using drugs**

  Why do you suppose people would use drugs in this way?

  Possible responses: to feel better; because they are addicted; they don't feel good enough about themselves to go without drugs; they are sick; they don't know what else to do; it's what everyone else does.

- **Consequences of using drugs**

  Does using drugs make people feel better?

  Look for responses suggesting that they may make people feel better for a little while, but over time people who use drugs feel worse.

  Is using drugs a healthy choice?

  Look for negative responses.

- **Ways people might take drugs**

  What are some ways people take these kinds of drugs?

  Possible responses: smoke, take pills, snort or sniff, drink, inject. If students do not volunteer "inject," bring it up and offer a description of injection drug use.

People who take certain kinds of drugs may use needles that let them put the drug directly into a vein (their blood system). They use the same kinds of needles you see in a doctor's office or clinic if you are getting a shot.

AIDS and Injection Drug Use

Describe the way the AIDS germ can be passed when people share injection drug needles and syringes. Following are the points to emphasize.

- **Sharing of needles**
  Sometimes, people who take drugs this way share needles and syringes. Because these needles and syringes are hard to get if you are not a doctor, people who take drugs with needles often have to use the same needle over and over, and may share the needles with other people.

- **Using drugs with needles is always dangerous**
  Using drugs with needles this way is always dangerous, for many reasons. One reason is that the drugs themselves are dangerous, and can make a person very sick.

  Another reason is that people who use needles and syringes illegally can get infections if the needles have been used before and are not absolutely germ-free.

- **People who share needles can get the AIDS germ**
  A person who shares needles might get the AIDS germ inside his or her body. Here's how that can happen. First, remember that the AIDS germ lives in blood. If someone puts drugs into his vein using a needle and syringe, he will get a little blood in the needle. Imagine that when he is done, he gives the needle and syringe to someone else to use.

  She also puts drugs into her vein using the needle and syringe. When she does this, a little of the blood from the first person is still in the needle. So she gets this person's blood in her body. If the first person had the AIDS germ in his blood, then the second person probably got the AIDS germ in her body too.

How AIDS Works: Grades K–3

Selected Resources

THERE ARE MANY MATERIALS currently available for elementary-age children and those who work with them on the topic of HIV and AIDS prevention. Following is a list of selected resources that may prove useful to you.

Books for Children

Alex, the Kid with AIDS. L. Gerard. 1990. Concept Book Series. Niles, IL: A. Whitman.

(Grades 2–5) This story is about a fourth grade boy with AIDS and how he and his schoolmates learn to deal with his illness. Alex learns how to make friends and to fit in, in spite of his disease. His classmates learn how HIV/AIDS differs from other diseases, how to protect themselves from transmission, and how to accept and have compassion for someone who has AIDS.

Daddy and Me. J. Moutoussamy-Ashe. 1993. New York: Alfred A. Knopf.

(Grades K–2) This book is a collection of photographs of Arthur Ashe and his daughter, after the tennis champion had been diagnosed with AIDS. Six-year-old daughter Camera talks about loving and living with a parent with AIDS.

Germ Smart: Children's Activities in Disease Prevention. J. Scheer. 1990. Santa Cruz, CA: ETR Associates.

(Grades K–3) This resource guide and activity book gives age-appropriate examples for teaching children about the basics of good hygiene, the immune system and self-esteem. Includes games, roleplays and puppetry.

The Immune System: Your Magic Doctor. H. Garvy. 1992. Los Gatos, CA: Shire Press.

(Grades 4–6) This book has colorful cartoon illustrations about the immune system and how it works. Based on the award-winning film of the same name, the book uses a fortress to illustrate the outside defenses of the immune system and an army of soldiers to depict the inner defenses. Includes information on how a child can help to stay healthy.

Jimmy and His Family. M. Tasker. 1992. The Association for the Care of Children's Health, 7910 Woodmont Ave., Suite 300, Bethesda, MD 20814, (301) 654-6549.

(Grades K–6) This story about what it's like to be a child with HIV should be read along with parents or teacher. Both English and Spanish translations are included.

Play Safe: Teaching Children Not to Play with Found Syringes. M. Williams, G. Savina and J. Vaccaro. 1990. Tacoma-Pierce County Health Department, 3629 South D Street, MS #152, Tacoma, WA 98408, (206) 591-6500.

(Grades K–2) Designed as a flip chart, this book has illustrations about syringes and safety on the front of each page and teacher's script on the back side. Could be used as part of a general safety unit.

Talking About Death: A Dialogue Between Parent and Child. E. Grollman. 1990. Boston: Beacon Press.

(Grades 3–6) To help children cope with death, this book features a parents' guide, an illustrated read-along story and a comprehensive resource section.

Touch Talk!, *Stop It!* and *Tell Someone!* ETR Associates, P.O. Box 1830, Santa Cruz, CA 95061, (800) 321-4407.

(Grades K–2, 3–4, 5–6) These booklets teach children what to do if someone touches them and they don't like it. To be read with parents.

What's a Virus, Anyway? The Kids' Book About AIDS. D. Fassler and K. McQueen. 1990. Burlington, VT: Waterfront Books.

(Grades K–5) Can be used to introduce AIDS to young children. Includes drawings and questions from children. Requires supplemental information on sexual transmission of AIDS. Best used by parents, or by teachers to introduce an AIDS education curriculum.

You and HIV: A Day at a Time. L. S. Baker. 1991. Elk Grove Village, IL: W. B. Saunders.

(Grades K–6) Encourages HIV-positive children to learn about, understand and take part in their illness and treatment. Best if read with parents.

Sexuality Education Curricula

Abstinence: Comprehensive Health for the Middle Grades. D. Zevin. 1996. Santa Cruz, CA: ETR Associates.

(Grades 6–8) Curriculum emphasizes that abstinence eliminates the risks of unwanted pregnancy, sexually transmitted disease and emotional upheavals. Promotes positive relationships without sexual intercourse and provides skill practice in communication, decision making and goal setting.

All About Life. C. Monastersky and E. Phillips-Angeles. 1995. Seattle-King County Department of Public Health, Family Planning Publications, 2124 4th Ave., Seattle, WA 98121, (206) 296-4672.

(Grades K–4) Seeks to build a foundation and enhance children's skills in communication, comprehension, awareness, decision making, sexuality and self-esteem. The program includes roleplaying, drawing and booklets to be read with parents designed to help increase partnerships between school and home.

F.L.A.S.H. (Family Life and Sexual Health). E. Reiss and P. Hillard. 1988. Seattle-King County Department of Public Health, Family Planning Publications,

2124 4th Ave., Seattle, WA 98121, (206) 296-4672.

(Grades 5–6) Based on "universal values": respect must be given for the individuality of the student and his or her peers; honest communication is fundamental in all relationships; people have a responsibility to learn as much as possible about themselves and others.

Growing Up and Learning to Feel Good About Yourself: An Educator's Bilingual Guide to Teaching Puberty. B. Petrich-Kelly and K. Rohm. 1996. ETR Associates, P.O. Box 1830, Santa Cruz, CA 95061, (800) 321-4407.

(Grades 5–6) English/Spanish curriculum provides accurate information about functions of the male and female reproductive systems, common puberty dilemmas and problem-solving strategies. These topics are covered in 3 general areas: self-awareness, self-protection and self-appreciation/self-esteem. The curriculum encourages young children to feel normal and natural about their sexuality.

Learning About Family Life: Resources for Learning and Teaching. B. Sprung. 1992. New York, NY: Bantam, Doubleday, Bell Publishing Group, The Education and Library Division.

(Grades K–3) Supports the concept that sex is pleasurable and that curiosity about one's body is natural and healthy. Based on 4 elements: interpersonal relationships; human growth, development, sexuality and reproduction; responsible personal behavior; and building strong families.

Postponing Sexual Involvement: An Educational Series for Preteens. M. Howard and M. Mitchell. 1995. Emory/Grady Teen Services Program, Grady Memorial Hospital, 80 Butler Street, Atlanta, GA 30335.

(Grades 5–6) Developed to help preteens learn the skills of resisting pressure to become sexually involved before they are ready. Five sessions present information and activities related to (1) societal pressures to becoming sexually active, (2) risks of early sexual behavior, (3) peer pressure, (4) assertiveness techniques, and (5) reinforcement in using new skills.

When I'm Grown. Advocates for Youth. 1992/3. Advocates for Youth, 1025 Vermont Ave. NW, Washington, DC 20005, (202) 347-5700.

(Grades K–2, 3–4, 5–6) Each of three volumes has age-appropriate activities, group discussions, worksheets, games and take-home projects. Volume 1 (grades K–2) discusses cultural diversity and uses roleplaying about being a parent. Volume 2 (grades 3–4) addresses finding one's individual strengths (self-esteem), and includes roleplaying about sexual touch and abuse. Volume 3 (grades 5–6) focuses on communicating about sexuality with parents and identifying risky behavior in dating.

Videos for Children

A Is for AIDS. 1992. 15 minutes. The Altschul Group, 1560 Shuman Ave., Suite 100, Evanston, IL 60201, (800) 323-9084.

(Grades K–6) Talking animated dog

explains AIDS to 3 young children. Interviews 2 children (a 9-year-old girl and Ryan White) who have AIDS. Mentions sex and drugs without expanding or clarifying transmission in detail. Depicts immune system in cartoon format.

AIDS: A Different Kind of Germ. 1991. 16 minutes. ETR Associates, P.O. Box 1830, Santa Cruz, CA. 95061. (800) 321-4407.

(Grades K–3) Excellent video that blends live action and animation to explain the effect of AIDS on the body's immune system. Straightforward and factual, the program dispels many common fears and misconceptions. With the help of a young girl named Tracy and her cartoon friend, Microscopic Mike, kids learn why the AIDS virus is different from other kinds of infections, and how adults and children are most commonly exposed.

A Conversation with Magic. 1992. 28 minutes. Magic Johnson Foundation, Inc., 2029 Century Park East, Suite 810, Los Angeles, CA 90067, (310) 785-0201.

(Grades 4–8) This televised program features basketball player Magic Johnson talking with a group of children about HIV/AIDS. Includes rap music about all the ways young people can and can't get HIV. Beside educating about the disease, there is discussion about supporting and respecting people who have AIDS. Available in Spanish, and in versions with or without mention of condoms.

Let's Talk About AIDS. 1992. 14 minutes. Human Relations Media, 175 Tompkins Ave., Pleasantville, NY 10570, (800) 431-2050.

(Grades 3–6) Includes an especially good segment showing HIV infected elementary school students. Presents 3 means of transmission but glosses over "safe sex," which is presented while the image of 2 children, a girl in a bridal gown and a boy in a tux, kiss each other. Some of the information is presented in rap which is somewhat confusing. Children are interviewed, but the information is presented as isolated facts.

Ryan White Talks to Kids About AIDS. 1990. 28 minutes. Film for the Humanities and Sciences, Inc., P.O. Box 2053, Princeton, NJ 08543, (800) 257-5126.

(Grades 5–8) Adapted from a national broadcast of the Phil Donahue Show. Ryan White offers insights and information about having AIDS and answers questions from an audience of teenagers and preteens. Ryan talks about the pain and humiliation of going to schools that did not want him and having schoolmates who had been told to avoid him. Information about AIDS epidemiology, transmission and prevention are given.

Thumbs Up for Kids: AIDS Education. 1990. 23 minutes. AIMS Media, 9710 DeSoto Ave., Chatsworth, CA 91311, (800) 367-2467

(Preschool/primary grades) Presented by Ruby Unger, a former Romper Room teacher. Upbeat and engaging, and young children and preschool and kindergarten teachers will enjoy it for that reason.

Main weakness is its neglect of any discussion of sexual transmission or injection drugs, and the emphasis on handwashing and demonstrations of germs being passed from child to child through casual transmission. Includes footage about HIV infected children.

What Is AIDS? 1995. 15 minutes. ETR Associates, P.O. Box 1830, Santa Cruz, CA, 95061-1830. (800) 321-4407.

(Grades 4–6) Children learn that with appropriate behavior, they have nothing to fear from the AIDS virus, or from people who have AIDS. Describes AIDS using a baseball analogy that may be confusing to children, with adults in costumes playing the immune system team against the germ team. Comes with a discussion guide.

What Kids Want to Know About Sex and Growing Up. 1992. 60 minutes. Children's Television Workshop. Available through Sesame Street retail stores, or call (510) 429-1515, ext. 248.

(Grades 4–6) A good presentation about puberty and sexuality. Aired on PBS, March, 1992. Designed to help parents discuss sexuality with children in a straightforward manner. Comes with parents' guide.

Materials for Adults

AIDS Prevention Guide: The Facts About HIV Infection and AIDS; Putting the Facts to Use. U.S. Department of Health and Human Services. 1994. CDC National AIDS Clearinghouse, P.O. Box 6003, Rockville, MD 20849-6003, (800) 458-5231.

Booklet discusses ways one can and cannot become HIV infected, and presents answers to common questions. Includes information on how to talk to children about HIV/AIDS at different age levels, from late elementary to high school. Has a section on how to organize a community response to AIDS.

Are You Sad Too? Helping Children Deal with Loss and Death. D. Seibert, J. Drolet and J. Fetro. 1993. Santa Cruz, CA: ETR Associates.

Book for teachers, parents and other caregivers of children up to age 10. Helps adults improve their communication and coping skills, critical for managing an immediate loss and preparing for a healthier future. Gives common questions with appropriate answers at each developmental stage.

Dictionary of AIDS-Related Terminology. J. Huber. 1993. New York, NY: Neal-Schumann Publisher, Inc.

Resource book includes definitions for over 1,000 common key words, names and phrases generally associated with discussion of HIV and AIDS. Includes abbreviations, acronyms, historical terms, key persons, organizations, medical terminology, drugs and therapies, and sources of HIV-related information.

Does AIDS Hurt? Educating Young Children About AIDS. M. Quackenbush and S. Villarreal. 1992. 2d Edition. Santa Cruz, CA: ETR Associates.

Book for teachers, parents and other

care providers of children up to age 10. Includes information, terminology and age-appropriate guidelines for educating young children about HIV and AIDS. Suggests effective ways to trouble shoot problems that might arise when discussing HIV/AIDS with young children.

Guidelines for Comprehensive Sexuality Education: Kindergarten–12th Grade. SIECUS (Sex Information and Education Council of the United States). 1991. SIECUS, 130 W. 42nd St., Suite 2500, New York, NY 10036, (212) 819-9770.

Set of guidelines developed by a task force of leading health, education and sexuality professionals. The guidelines provide a framework for educators and policymakers who want to design or evaluate a comprehensive sexuality education program. Divided into 4 developmental levels: early elementary, upper elementary, junior high or middle school, and high school.

HIV/AIDS: A Challenge to Us All. 1993. Pediatric AIDS Foundation, 1311 Colorado Avenue, Santa Monica, CA 90404.

(Parents of elementary school children) This teaching aid includes 2 videos, a leader's guide for parent meetings, and sample parent letters and questionnaires designed to stimulate discussion. The package is designed to inform parents about HIV in children and to allay fears about allowing their children to attend school or associate with children who have HIV or AIDS. The first video shows a school meeting where parents learn about HIV/AIDS and how it might or might not affect their children. The second video shows scenarios of parents talking to and answering questions from their children about HIV/AIDS. Also available in Spanish.

The HIV Challenge: Prevention Education for Young People. M. Quackenbush, K. Clark and M. Nelson, eds. 1995. 2d Edition. Santa Cruz, CA: ETR Associates.

Book includes 28 chapters by experts on HIV/AIDS education. Written for health educators of children in grades K–12. Covers designing, implementing and evaluating successful HIV/AIDS prevention programs. Includes ways to reach minority youth and special populations; age-appropriate prevention information; and discussion of religious, legal and medical issues.

HIV Education and Health Education in the United States: A National Survey of Local School District Policies and Practices. D. Holtzman, B. Z. Greene, G. C. Ingraham, L. A. Daily, D. G. Demchuk and L. J. Kolbe. 1992. American School Health Association, P.O. Box 708, Kent, OH 44240-0708, (216) 678-1601.

Report assesses the extent to which HIV and health education policies and practices are required by United States school districts. The grade levels at which HIV prevention education is required, curriculum content and supporting practices and policies are included.

HIV: Health Facts. L. Stang and K. Miner. 1994. Santa Cruz, CA: ETR Associates.

Educators' resource book explains

infection through illness and death; discusses how HIV attacks the body and the body's response; and examines transmission and testing for HIV. Also covers risk and prevention behaviors.

HIV: Talking with Your Child. ETR Associates, P.O. Box 1830, Santa Cruz, CA, 95061-1830. (800) 321-4407.

Pamphlet for parents offers specific advice on how and when to begin talking to children about HIV/AIDS. Includes basic guidelines for talking, plus age-appropriate suggestions for talking about HIV.

How Can I Tell You? Secrecy and Disclosure with Children When a Family Member Has AIDS. M. Tasker. 1992. Association for the Care of Children's Health, 7910 Woodmont Ave., Suite 300, Bethesda, MD 20814, (301) 654-6549.

Through the use of discussion and family stories, this book provides a sensitive approach to the many complex and changing issues around disclosing an HIV diagnosis to a child.

Responding to HIV and AIDS. J. Burger, ed. 1992. National Education Association Health Information Network, 1201 16th St. NW, Washington, DC 20036, (202) 822-7570.

Booklet written for teachers and health educators seeks to educate and allay fears about HIV transmission in the school setting. Includes basic information about HIV/AIDS, plus a section on the proper handling of body fluids when someone is ill or injured. Another section addresses how to show compassion and help people who have HIV or AIDS.

School-Based HIV Prevention: A Multidisciplinary Approach. D. Kerr, D. Allensworth and J. Gayle. 1991. American School Health Association, P.O. Box 708, Kent, OH 44240-0708, (216) 678-1601.

Book for school personnel and policymakers is based on the assumption that an effective program must include planning and activities that incorporate policy, instruction (with media support), role modeling, peer education, direct intervention, environmental change and evaluation. Includes a chapter on what skills students need for preventing HIV infection.

Sex: Talking with Your Child. ETR Associates, P.O. Box 1830, Santa Cruz, CA, 95061-1830. (800) 321-4407.

Pamphlet for parents discusses how and when to raise the topic of sexuality to young children. Gives suggestions on how to deal with sensitive situations and includes basic information on sexual development of children from birth to age 6.

Talking with Kids About AIDS: A Program for Parents and Other Adults Who Care. J. Tiffany, D. Tobias, A. Raqib and J. Ziegler. 1991. Ithaca, NY: Cornell University, Media Services.

Program for parents and other caring adults is designed to enhance communication skills and encourage confidence as educators for the young people in their lives. Provides information on risk assessment and risk reduction and includes a teaching guide, resource manual and communication handbook.

Talking with Your Child About a Troubled World. L. S. Dumas. 1992. New York: Fawcett Columbine.

Book for parents of preschool through preteen children offers 16 general guidelines for talking about serious subjects with children and discusses more than a dozen critical social issues, including AIDS, racism, war, natural disasters, divorce and homelessness. Each chapter includes a resource list of helpful organizations and books about the subject being discussed.

When Sex Is the Subject: Attitudes and Answers for Young Children. P. Wilson. 1991. Santa Cruz, CA: ETR Associates.

Book for teachers, parents and other care providers of children up to age 10. Provides a general discussion of sexuality education and childhood development. Shows how to use a positive, reassuring attitude to discuss sexuality. Gives age-appropriate answers to children's common questions about sexuality.